DR. NINA
AND THE PANTHER

DR. NINA
AND THE PANTHER

Shirley P. Wheeler

DODD, MEAD & COMPANY, NEW YORK

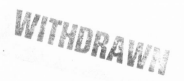

Copyright © 1976 by Shirley P. Wheeler
Printed in the United States of America
by The Haddon Craftsmen, Inc., Scranton, Penna.

Library of Congress Cataloging in Publication Data

Wheeler, Shirley P
  Dr. Nina and the panther.

  1. Price, Nina Mae, 1882–1974. 2. Women
physicians—Pennsylvania—Biography. 3. Monroe
Co., Pa.—Biography. I. Title.
R154.P8627W48   616.8'55'00924 [B]   76–25814
ISBN 0-396-07348-4

...Acknowledgments

For allowing me to search their memories, I thank my sisters, Bobby Westbrook, Carol Sams, and Catharine Velkoff; for various kinds of help, both practical and supportive, I acknowledge a debt to Louise J. Williams, Albert Chaiken, and Joseph S. Evans, Jr.; for his professional skill, I am grateful to William Whipple, editor. I give special thanks to Christopher Wheeler, Linda Lester, and Robin Torrey, who always knew their grandmother's story needed telling.

.

PART
ONE

"Lord in the morning"

In a late summer of the mid-1890s two little children walked up a dusty mountain road. Not a leaf stirred. The slanting sun was yellow where it broke through the thick overhang of branches to speckle the wagon trail, but was fiercely white on the slabs of limestone that, convoluted and exposed at the tops of the rises, forced the trees back to better footing away from the road. The children walked quietly, without speaking, their bare feet soundless in the locust-buzzing, bird-calling, squirrel-chattering forest.

Anyone who might have been watching the children would have known they were not mountain-bred. These children, one nine years old, the other six, walked with their backs straight, their two dark, shapely heads carried lightly, with grace. Someone, hours ago, had braided the hair on each narrow skull with such skill and care that even in the late afternoon the neat plaits still pulled the delicate skin over the temples up and back, giving each set of eyes a slanty, exotic charm.

There was, however, no one to watch the children—no one at all. The scattered farms that struggled to keep little cleared patches unreclaimed by the central Pennsylvania forests were miles from each other and miles from the road. The children were alone and on their way home. Home was a tent near the top of the mountain. Each child carried a full pail of wild berries. It would have been obvious that in spite of their dusty feet, their bramble-scratched arms, their weariness, their silence, they walked with an air of pensiveness and responsibility that is always the mark of prematurely civilized children. But there was no one to watch them or to judge their quality.

They were entirely alone as they rounded a curve over a ridge and came face to face with a panther lying on the white, hot rocks slanting across the road. A panther is a mountain lion, a puma, a great wild, tawny lion-without-a-mane, with the shoulder-muscle development of a leopard, with the lean flanks and pulled-up belly of a jaguar. This panther's back was to the sun, and the shadow of his great, blunt head was purple on the bleached rocks. The children stood frozen in horror, their sun-struck eyes blank with surprise. The panther's great yellow eyes opened wider in interest and mild alarm. The locusts, in the strange phenomenon that happens now and then for an instant, stopped all their noise at once. No leaf stirred.

Just for a moment, we'll leave the three of them there, frozen in time. You must believe that the children will save themselves somehow because one of them, the elder, grew up to be my mother.

She grew up to be many other things and many other children's mother, too. This child facing the panther also grew up to be panther-prone; that is to say, she was so vigorous and so full of life force that she did not fear death, and so single-minded in pursuing each goal as it appeared that she did not give consideration even to danger until it stared her in the face with the bright eyes of a Nemesis.

I wonder how other people feel about their mothers. Once in a while, when the situation is such as to make the question not exactly impertinent, I ask, but I always get a silly answer. Dear Old Mom always turns out to be a hard worker and a good mother, considering everything; she is always loved in a comfortable fashion that is perilously close to indifference. This is not the attitude that makes strong men dying on the battlefield or in their peaceful beds cry out, "Mother! Mother!" Not the name of the be-

loved wife or the name of a child, but "Mother! Save Me!"
Surely the bond between child and mother is vastly less
casual than Good Old Mom for people other than me. And
why does the bond run only from child to mother and not
run also the other way? Even when my mother, old, old as
she was, and sick, and not always in the real world, at the
end of her life, cried out in her sleep, she called to *her*
mother. Not to her truly loved second husband, not to her
children, but to her mother, who, ninety years before on
that Pennsylvania mountain, loved her without tenderness
and rejected her without compassion. Why is the bond
from child to mother a one-way street?

But we have left the children frozen in terror under the
August sun, staring into the eyes of a panther. What will
they do? Everyone knows instinctively that to stare into the
eyes of an animal, human or otherwise, is to establish an
immediate, meaningful relationship that can be disastrous.
Those who love expose their eyes; those who are artists at
deceit practice the direct, open, candid gaze. For everyone
else, there is an atavistic avoidance of the fixed stare. We
know better, without having to learn. The first thing the
older child did was to say to her little sister, "Don't look
at him." The little one's eyeballs swiveled away toward the
trees, although her neck was too rigid with fright to turn
with them. The older child, looking only at the shadow of
the panther's head, slowly shifted her bucket of berries into
her left hand, her right hand groping and finding her little
sister's hand. There was no way to retreat. Such a beast
could outrun a deer. There was no help anywhere on the
road behind. "God will save us," she said. "Sing!" From
somewhere she had remembered an old saying that a wild
animal will never attack a singing human. Or did she remember? My mother was forever making up old sayings as
though she had a private pipeline into the prehistoric hu-

man past. "Sing," she said, and started singing herself, her voice thin and tight.

"There is sunshine in my soul today," she sang, her sister joining her in a voice little more than a whisper. Together, hand in hand, the older one in the lead, they walked straight toward the panther.

"Oh, there is sunshine, blessed sunshine
When the peaceful happy moments roll,"

they sang as they passed the wild beast, who had risen to his feet. His warm breath on the older child's shoulder caused her to give him one glance that took in only the bright bits of straw caught in his lion-brown fur.

"When Jesus shows his shining face
There is sunshine in my soul."

And they were past. On they marched, singing the second verse.

I am exasperated with myself to feel prickles of laughter inside at the fact that they sang the second verse of a hymn. If this were fiction, I would never have thought of a second verse, but when you have heard how these children came to be on a far mountain with their beautiful, stern-faced, gray-eyed mother, it will not seem incongruous that they knew the second verse and, indeed, all the verses to all the evangelical hymns. Meanwhile, they are in mortal danger and there is nothing funny about mortal danger. I think I laugh inside because a sense of humor is the first defense of the true coward and, in the face of raw courage, what can cowards do but prickle with wondering amusement while taking thought to avoid the places where panthers might lie in wait?

So the children marched ahead, now singing strongly, the panther somewhere behind them. The road up to the next turning must have seemed endless. They dared not look back. The very act of turning to look at danger paralyzes the will. They marched around the turn and, as soon as they could assume they were out of sight of those blazing yellow eyes, they ran. They ran so fast that the prints of their little toes made long blurs in the dusty road and the berries from the pails in their frantic hands scattered in all directions. Over the next ridge they came upon a wagon loaded with firewood, the farmer standing up behind his horse, his eyes popping from their sockets.

"God almighty, kids! I seen a great big painter jump to the woods. He musta been followin' you. Lucky I come," he said. My mother remembered his name for ninety years; salvation, thy name is John Hurd! John Hurd turned his nervous horse, who had also seen the "painter," and took the children to the tent where their mother waited without fear, knowing that Jesus saves. John Hurd went off to gather the mountain farmers together to hunt down the first panther to be seen in the central Pennsylvania woods for thirty years. The beast was tracked and killed the next night. He measured eight feet three inches from nose to tail. May John Hurd be driving an untroubled horse over the golden streets of Heaven!

...2

What were they doing there, the children? And why were they with their mother in a tent? We have to know these things. I will tell them quickly because the era of America behind my mother is history and, no matter how fascinating that slice of history may be, it is a time unlit for me by the handed-down accounts that illuminate my mother's lifetime.

The children's mother, Harriet, was the only child of an

English couple who had emigrated to the United States. Her father was a younger son of minor English nobility, but since oldest sons of major noble families felt no call to emigrate to the New World, this minor son held a position in Philadelphia society that many Main Line families today would envy. He was a well-to-do Victorian and a snob. Two younger sisters came from England to visit him. Both married Americans, one to remain in Philadelphia, the other to "go west" with her husband to establish a woolen mill in a small town near Williamsport, Pennsylvania. To that town, which they naturally named after themselves, their niece Harriet often came to spend the summer. The town still exists today and, as far as I know, their descendents still manufacture fine English-style woolens.

Back in Philadelphia, sixteen-year-old, beautiful Harriet fell in love and eloped with a young blacksmith. What could a good Victorian father do in those days but cross the name of his only child out of the family Bible, execute a new will leaving his estate to his two sisters, and with his broken-hearted wife live a life of emotional deprivation? This he did, and both of Harriet's parents died before they were fifty years old. "How are they brought into desolation, as in a moment."

When my mother could be prodded into recounting to strangers we had brought home some of the adventures of her childhood, she often spoke of her father as a "mechanical engineer." This was largely a lie; Harriet's husband was a blacksmith, a happy blacksmith who, at fourteen, had lied his way into the Union Army to serve for the last year of the Civil War as a drummer boy. When Mark Case married Harriet, he was twenty-one. He was a beautiful blacksmith, six feet four, with crisp, curling black hair and bright blue eyes. He loved to laugh, to sing, and to work with his hands. What more could a willful, highly tutored Philadelphia debutante want?

They fled Philadelphia to go west—to the real West where the cowboys were, and the Pony Express, and Indians, and gold. This was the era in our country when manual labor was vastly more valuable than all of little Harriet's Latin and Greek and History of Art, so their flight was more of a stagger away from the East Coast. Their problem was not how to go on west but how to extricate themselves from the clinging hands that intended to hold fast to a young man who could forge horseshoes, mend wagons, weld pipes, and devise ingenious ways to repair broken parts of newfangled machinery. It's a wonder they even got as far as they did, which was Michigan.

In the little town of Ithaca, Michigan, they settled, in part because Harriet was pregnant and in part because the town's blacksmith had just gone away with the gold rush. It must have been a vigorous little place. Two-thirds of the population were under thirty years old, and the industrial revolution that was convulsing western Europe and the American east coast was already making itself felt in miniature, usable, happy ways in Ithaca. Everyone who was not yet anyone was importing machinery that had no spare parts and that was only dimly understood. What scope for a young man who had a feel for mechanical things! Maybe he *was* a "mechanical engineer." Lies told by a real raconteur are often more than half-truths.

Harriet bore eight children in fifteen years, and a final child, the ninth, three years later. Of all these children, only two remained with her, Nina and Dorothy, the two who sang their way past the panther.

John, the oldest child, left home at age sixteen to go on west. The great winds of the age were blowing children away from their parents, always westward. John lived to an old, old age but never once wrote to his parents. He was as lost to them as though he had died.

Jessie, the second child, married at sixteen with her parents' consent. Jessie evidently was not much liked by her parents. They allowed her to marry a young farmer and then dropped her the way one drops an acquaintance whom one finds uninteresting. Maybe when one has eight children one does not feel compelled to like them all. I met Aunt Jessie many years later. We arrived late at night because we had trouble finding the lonely place the two old people were farming. They were waiting for us, long past their bedtime, and the grotesque shadows on the walls made by the flaring oil lamps were frightening to a city child. I wonder why her parents dropped her so casually. She had a quality that should have been worth care, an inner warmth that was shyer and more tender than my mother's intensity, but recognizable. She was having trouble with dentures and kept her store teeth in her mouth only long enough to kiss us all and make a good first impression on the sister she had never really known. But she had pinned a brave little red bow in her snow-white hair, and her faded blue eyes looked upon us all with such a shy, diffident, timid glow that I stopped being afraid of the shadows. Her husband must have loved her still to stay up so late for strangers. "When thy father and mother forsake thee, then the Lord will take thee up."

The next four children died all at once in a diphtheria epidemic. We are now so accustomed to immunization that the very idea of four children dying all at once in one beautiful spring season, when the apple blossoms are bursting the trees and the little lambs are leaping stiff-legged in the meadow, is offensive. But in the old days it was not inconceivable, it was not unexpected. Maybe that's why no matter how many children one had in those days, one didn't "relate" too closely, one didn't care too much, one didn't overmanage any one child's life. One planned ahead to love and lose and keep on living. One after the other, some within hours of others, Joe, Claudia, Clyde, and Ivus died. During this time of crisis, Nina, six years old, was put in charge of her three-year-old sister. She played with Dorothy outside in the fresh spring air. She was bewildered that the vigorous, exciting world of a large family of children could disappear so suddenly, and she was without any real comprehension that death was busily folding up that world and filing it neatly away underground.

Harriet, the mother, held up well under disaster. Perhaps, though, this was the beginning of the change in her personality and goals that culminated in a lonely tent on a far mountain, but no one could be sure. We can be sure that no one changes overnight. The boulder that tips from its bed has already been undermined by many freezes, many thaws, and the final push by wind, water, or gentle tremor only seems to be the force that made it move and crash and change in some measure the face of the earth. By a similar erosion in the human sphere, the disintegration of personality can progress in small rents and rifts until suddenly the psychic fabric tears apart and only by looking back do we think we know where the first signs of the disaster began. Maybe, for Harriet, it began here. Or perhaps it began a year before when she heard of the death of her parents. I can't believe that she minded terribly that they were dead. The rash people of the world have a happy knack of substituting one relationship for another when what they do cuts them off from those who love them and oppose them. But it might have been a blow to her that they didn't leave her the money; the reckless ones of the world often have, oddly enough, more cupidity in their hearts than the prudent. Those whom they discard are expected to cherish and remember and forgive without rancor, and often they do, but Harriet's parents took their hard hearts with them into their stony Victorian graves. "Can a woman forget her sucking child?" asks Isaiah. "Yea, they may forget," he answers himself. It must have been a shock.

Whenever the change in Harriet's personality began, it was not yet visible to those closest to her. She was strong and comforting and willing to be comforted. She was also pregnant with her final child, and to be pregnant is to be shielded against absolute despair.

The baby was born three months later and he died within three months of cholera infantum. And now the change came. Harriet was fragmented by grief, resentment, bewilderment. She refused to be comforted and, in fact, refused to be there at all. She sat idle and unresponsive, looking out the window over the flat Michigan fields; she would talk to no one. She didn't care who was hungry or cold or sad. Neither her husband nor the children could reach her. Like Lot's wife, she was a pillar of salt, tearless.

One beautiful November day, sixty-five years later, I heard the story from my mother under rather odd circumstances. After my sisters and I had grown up and married, we came home when we could, partly to see Mother and partly to eat. Dr. Nina was a great natural gourmet cook. She had trained her hired help in the basics of cooking, but she would rush in at the last minute from her medical rounds to add the final wine, spices, seasoning, butter, cream, or lavish handfuls of dewy mountain huckleberries picked that morning by a grateful patient. The hot breads, sturdy meats, delicate vegetables, and tender greens were worth coming hundreds of miles to eat.

But in order to have any time to talk to Mother, whoever was visiting had to go with her on her calls. Her medical practice was widespread and she cared about her patients. After one middle-of-the-night baby delivery, we were riding home together about eight o'clock in the morning. The

Indian summer sky was already a bright, warm blue and the Pocono Mountains were shouting with color. We pulled to the side of the road to look over a blazing valley and Mother said, almost to herself, "It was a morning just like this when my mother's baby died."

I was startled. "Your mother's baby?" I asked.

"Yes," she said, still more to herself than to me. "She wouldn't believe we cared. I loved the baby, too, but she wouldn't believe me," and tears showered down her face.

I was horrified. I'd never seen my mother cry before. She cried all at once, like a child, so fresh was the grief and pain in the six-year-old hiding still under sixty-five more years of living.

I never saw her cry again. On that first Indian summer day long ago in Michigan, she knew, the way children sense what is real, that when her mother's baby died, the loss for them all was irretrievable.

...3

Several weeks after Harriet's baby died, Nina sat lonely and chilled on the chip pile. In the olden days of no central heating, every house had a chip pile in the yard. It was made by the chips that flew from the logs when they were split for firewood. The chips were used for kindling, but there were increasingly more chips than uses for them, so the pile grew during the winter. Chip piles were good to sit on, being fragrant and buoyant. Nina must have looked forlorn because a strange voice asked, "What's the matter, little girl? Why are you so sad?"

Nina turned to look up into the plain, kind face of a strange woman.

"I'm Mrs. Squires," the lady said. "I'm a new neighbor.

What's the matter?"

"My mother's baby died and she won't talk to me."

"Well, maybe she'll talk to me," the lady said. "Maybe I can help. Let's try." And she walked to the back door, knocked, turned the knob, and walked in.

Inside, she stood looking for a moment at the woman by the window. "Your baby isn't dead, Mrs. Case, he is only sleeping," she said. Harriet turned, startled and shocked.

"Please, please don't misunderstand me," Mrs. Squires said. "I only want to tell you the Truth. I think you have always believed that when anyone dies, the soul immediately enters Heaven or Hell while the body lies buried in the grave. This is not true. Your darling little one sleeps peacefully in the grave until Jesus comes; then He bids him come forth, and sends His angels to bear him safely to your arms, and you will look down into the face of your beautiful baby. He will grow up with you in Heaven. Heaven is a real place and we will be real people looking exactly as we do now. We will build houses and inhabit them; we will plant vineyards and eat the fruit thereof; we shall walk and not be weary; we shall run and not faint; and there shall be naught that can hurt or destroy; neither shall there be any more pain. Let me sit down and I will prove it to you." She drew a Bible from under her apron, and for two hours she read and explained from the Bible "the state of the dead."

Whatever events contributed to the alteration of Harriet's personality and whenever the change actually began, Mrs. Squires was to serve as the catalyst that brought about a new focus for Harriet's actions. Because of Mrs. Squires, the explosion occurred which was to tear the family apart and send Harriet and her two children to a tent on a high mountain for three years of summer heat and bitter winter snow. It would be comforting to blame Mrs. Squires or the particular religious sect for whom she was an apostle, but

Mrs. Squires was a kind woman whose way was paved with good intentions and we cannot blame the Seventh-Day Adventist Church any more than we can blame any church for the excessive zeal of its converts.

And Harriet herself was, by temperament, excessive. I'll be glad to get rid of Harriet, because she threatens by her excess of zeal in whatever she does to take over my story. The life of a fanatic doesn't make a good story. Great fanatics take their places in history; little ones like Harriet walk the midnight halls, wringing their hands and crying to be justified. If Harriet wants her story told, she'll have to find someone else to tell it. But we can't get rid of Harriet until after she discards my mother the way one plucks off burrs from one's sleeve after a hike in the woods.

Maybe we should blame Mark, the handsome, happy blacksmith. We all know in our secret hearts that what we want most for ourselves is physical beauty, which almost none of us have. But true physical beauty often is accompanied by an insensitivity of spirit that blandly assumes an exemption from the onerous obligation of endearing oneself to others by tolerance and loving-kindness and diffidence. Mark was a blithe spirit, and tragedy left him still able to laugh and sing and work with his hands. Harriet's months of dumb misery may have been the careful gathering up of a wild resentment designed to make her husband suffer the death of spirit she herself had known. Mark remained intact under stress; he turned his exuberant joy in living away from grief and toward his remaining children. Harriet had never been physically demonstrative with any of the children; it was Mark who held and rocked and sang to them. In an almost pathetic effort to give to a few the love that had been spread among many, he drew Nina closer to him than any of the lost children had ever been. The more unreachable Harriet became, the more he tried to compensate to Nina and Dorothy for their shared rejection.

Certainly Harriet knew that Mark was fanatical in his distaste for the evangelical sects that were popping up out of the ground like crocuses. Of all the evangelical sects, Mark hated the "Advents" most. They not only took religion out of the churchhouse (where it belonged) and preached strange disciplines up and down the streets (where pleasant patterns were already in working order), but also expected momentarily the second coming of Christ and the end of the world, and therefore took a feckless attitude toward the value of personal possessions and a harsh view of the innocent pleasures of this world. Harriet, who knew of Mark's rejection of the Advents, successfully deceived him for months and months as he rejoiced in her reentrance into the everyday world. When all was discovered, more than a year later, Harriet was a confirmed Advent herself and was determined that Mark should follow wherever she might lead, or be left behind totally alone.

He found out what was going on behind his back by accident. He must have vaguely noticed that some new element had taken over his household. Often when he came home, Mrs. Squires, with her kind, apologetic, propitiating smile, would be fading out of the back door. Harriet started using strange terminology, such as "in these last days," "sign of the times," and "the sure word of prophecy," none of which sounded terribly Episcopalian. He must have noticed, because about midway between the time of innocent hope and final disaster, he asked, "Aren't you getting a little too deep into this religious stuff? You can't become a nun, you know, because you have us!" And he laughed.

Couldn't she, just? That laugh was to be wiped from his handsome face before he was many months older. "All flesh is grass, and all the goodliness thereof is as the flower of the field: The grass withereth."

A new character then entered the little family circle, by

way of the back door. The Elder Adam T. Bates began to slip in and out with Mrs. Squires. He was an ordained minister, the man from the home office who gets the signature on the binding contract. He studied with Harriet Coming Events, and Separation from the World, and Divine Healing. He could find, with a flip of Bible pages, the solution to any human problem. And it was the visits of Elder Bates that were to start a chain of gossip that Mark was the last to hear.

Mark had been improvising some machinery repair at the local mill and had finished early in the afternoon. He decided to go home. On the way home he met a neighbor, Jack Fink, whom he invited over with his wife that night for a sing. "We haven't seen you folks for months," Mark said.

"No," said Jack Fink, "and you won't see us, I'm afraid. My wife won't go to a house that Advent preacher has taken over with his flock." Poor kind Mrs. Squires had grown into a flock. She would have been astonished.

Mark was furious. He strode home and into the house before Elder Bates and Mrs. Squires could fade out of the back door. My mother was to remember only once, many years later, the words he used then. They were new words to her, and Mark, in a black rage, used them coldly and cruelly as he backed Elder Bates step by step out of the house, past the chip pile, and through the garden gate.

...4

The Seventh-Day Adventist Church of this story was an offshoot of the Great Advent Movement of nineteenth-century America. The movement held its first Camp Meeting in 1842 and set April 1844 for the second coming of

Christ. This date had been carefully calculated from Biblical prophecy. After much preparation and sacrifice and selling of property by the faithful, the world didn't end in April after all and a new date, recalculated to expel arithmetical error, was announced. October 22, 1844, was to be the day the world ended. During the entire year so much excitement and attraction were engendered that the established churches were forced to turn their attention to what they labeled "wild fanaticism" and to expel those of their members who expected the world to end in 1844. One of the more regular American Protestant churches announced that it felt "constrained to regard the Great Advent Movement as among the erroneous and strange doctrines which we are pledged to banish and drive away." In spite of this, converts flocked to the movement. During 1844 twenty-five Camp Meetings were held throughout the country, involving more than half a million people. I don't know what the population of the United States was in 1844, but half a million people preparing to leave this world can be an unsettling factor in the economy of any era.

The world didn't end in October, either, and after this second disappointment the Great Advent Movement fell apart. Remnants formed into other groups around other leaders. Most of the converts went home. One group formed itself into the Seventh-Day Adventist Church, which preached the second coming of Christ as imminent but not tied to any specific date. The belief of the Seventh-Day Adventists was that the world was in "the last days" foreseen by the prophets, and although the last days could endure for many, many years, they *could* be at their close. Today could be the last day, today!

The Seventh-Day Adventist Church in that era was Judaistic in its ritual—the Old Testament Jewish religion with Christ grafted on. Saturday was the seventh day, the

Sabbath; pork was unclean; certain foods could not be eaten in the same meal with other foods; no work, including cooking, should be done on the Sabbath. And most of all, the cry of the Jewish prophets was heard in the land: Repent! Repent!

The Seventh-Day Adventist Church also embraced a totally new set of doctrines promulgated by a new leader, Ellen White. Mrs. White and her followers believed her writings to be divinely inspired. All of the fundamentalist sects of that day, in fact, believed with Swedenborg that thought was not created, but was received from a source extraneous to the mundane sphere. Mrs. White gave a new and important element to the Judaic tenets of this church: an immediate, direct, and practical concern for the health of the human body. The dietary laws of the Jews were not, for Mrs. White, good enough, because they didn't go far enough. To her, the body was a medium through which the mind and soul are developed and made acceptable to God. Ill health and unbridled appetites corrupt. What one eats determines one's health, and only through perfect health can one control one's baser passions. Butter, cheese, meat, condiments, spices, coffee, tea, salt, alcohol—all these and more fevered the blood and weakened moral and intellectual powers. Moreover, guilt from sin diseased the mind, and a sick mind produced a sick body. In the light of present-day concern with cholesterol and psychosomatic illness, there is little in these tenets that is, in itself, strange.

What seems strange and interesting is that while, in the same era, Mary Baker Eddy was founding her Christian Science church, based on the doctrine that all illness was a result of erroneous human conception of God's perfect plan, that all medicine was useless and sinful as a substitute for correct thinking, another woman, our Ellen White, accepted disease as an outcome of a faulty understanding of

the God-given human body, which functioned well only
when imbibing the food God meant to be eaten—grain,
fruit, vegetables, nuts, and cold, pure water. She was more
than respectful of medicine and the training of competent
medical doctors who could treat the sick by aiding nature
in its work through diet, exercise, rest, and cleanliness.
Since healing was, to her, linked with the forgiveness of
sins, doctors were needed who could heal both mind and
body together. Herbal medicinal products, medical training, courage, hope, faith, and love all together could promote health and prolong life. In the same era, another
interesting woman, Amelia Bloomer, the great feminist,
evolved a female costume that she believed was in accord-
ance with the ideas of Mrs. White. But Mrs. White found
bloomers immodest and adopted a dress length that just
cleared the street. A lot of women were very busy in those
days.

Mrs. White's church, with its combination of bland vege-
tarian diet, Old Testament observances and rituals, and the
imminent second coming of Christ, was an impossible bill
of goods to sell to Mark Case. Mark's instinctive acceptance
of man's place in the animal kingdom was no part of Ellen
White's theology, nor was her insistence on the suppres-
sion and, indeed, eventual elimination of "animal propensi-
ties" any part of his.

In 1854 the Seventh-Day Adventist Church began holding modest tent meetings, single tents set up in small towns
or in open country. The preacher visited around during the
day. He helped with farmwork, leading the conversation
around to Bible themes. He asked pay for his farmwork.
The money he earned went to support tent living.

In 1868 the Seventh-Day Adventist Church held its first
full-scale Camp Meeting, organized on the pattern of the
Great Advent Movement's Camp Meetings, which col-

lapsed in 1844. The first new Camp Meeting had an encampment of twenty-two family tents and two large tents for services. This kind of Camp Meeting continued every summer until, suddenly, one of them involved our unhappy little family. In addition to the revived Camp Meeting technique, a new device was developed, the establishment of Bible workers. These were lay members of the congregation who visited homes and personally conducted Bible studies, answering questions and probing into personal problems that could never be considered at general meetings. So here we are with the threads in our hands that, put together, constitute the exact situation in which Harriet was zealously enmeshed.

The last year the family spent together must have been terrible. The frightening, improbable, and difficult events that followed could not have been, all together, so depressing and bewildering as the final year. After Elder Adam T. Bates had been backed out of the garden gate, Harriet began to have dreadful attacks of asthma. This was frightening for Mark and the children. Even worse, whenever Mark came into the house, Harriet would sit down, open the Bible, and read aloud. How exasperating for Mark! Every conversation between the parents turned into a dogmatic argument. Mark wanted eight-year-old Nina to go to school. Nina desperately wanted to go to school. Since her mother's baby died, Nina had had almost complete charge of her younger sister, and although she had long since learned to read and write, and read widely in her mother's extensive library, she dreamed of going to school the way a prisoner waits for the day that ends his sentence. Nina longed to be part of the life of the children she could watch from her fenced garden—games and laughter and tears she remembered from the time before her older brothers and sisters disappeared.

"No," Harriet said. "Nina will not go to school. She will stay home and continue her studies with me. She must not learn all the worldly things they teach in school. 'Be ye not unequally yoked together with unbelievers.' The children at school are children of the world and my children must not be influenced. Besides, she is already far ahead of children her own age, and I need her at home to help me with Dorothy." The door was closed and locked in the little prisoner's face.

Poor prisoner. What is so pathetic to me is that after the next three bitter years on the mountain, the child who never chose the path of righteousness was to be given to the church the way one casually puts a coin in the collection plate, while the mother, leaving the Seventh-Day Adventist Church, fled back to her Philadelphia beginnings and dwindled away into an uneventful old age, never to do a strange or brave act again, so far as I know.

The most acrimonious argument revolved around Harriet's insistence that they sell the blacksmith shop, their house, and most of their possessions and go to the mountains of central Pennsylvania that she had known and loved as a child. Mark was astonished. "But Harriet! All our life is here—our home, our friends, our graves. It's foolishness. I can't agree to folly."

"I want to be there when Jesus comes," Harriet declared. "You could find work anywhere and we won't need much. All these earthly things will be burned up anyway, when Jesus comes. 'I will lift up mine eyes unto the hills, from whence cometh my help.' "

Mark raged. "If it weren't for those interfering, sneaking, hell-born Advents, you wouldn't be such a fool!"

Harriet opened her Bible and read aloud.

The final battle between Harriet and Mark raged over Harriet's intention to go to Lock Haven, Pennsylvania, in

July, for a Seventh-Day Adventist Camp Meeting. This
was, she said, the least he could agree to let her do. Mark's
patience and temper, stretched too thin, snapped.

"All right," he said, "Go. But if you do, you can never
come back. I'm through. That goddamn church can take
care of you all."

"The Lord will provide," said Harriet. "We can no
longer stay here where God's name is taken in vain." One
up for Harriet!

Nina was given the choice of going with her mother and
sister or staying with her father. How strange it is that
when adults are enthusiastically biting on the bitter fruit
of discord, it is the teeth of the children that are set on edge.

"I'll have to go with Mother," she said. "What would she
do when she gets asthma without me?" The Lord provides
in very mysterious ways, and the fires of Harriet's zeal
were to be stoked and tended and enabled to burn because
of the decision of a small girl to provide for her mother.

Mark said, "She wouldn't have asthma if she hadn't taken
up with that goddamn religion." One up for Mark!

Harriet and the children left the next week, Harriet driving the horse and wagon on the long trip from Michigan
to Lock Haven, Pennsylvania. All they took with them in
the wagon were clothes, home-canned fruits and vegetables, a cooking pot, three light blankets, and books. Hundreds and hundreds of books. Mark had been so proud of
Harriet's erudition that, in the happier days, he had sent
for books, gone to cities for books, bought books from west-
ering families, rebound shabby books in soft home-tanned
cowhide and deerskin. He had built cherry-wood book-
shelves from floor to ceiling in every room of their little
home. Harriet took the books, leaving Mark the empty
shelves and an empty life. I can't believe his life was empty
for long, although what he did with it is unknown. My

mother never saw or heard of him again until she found his grave, years after he had died, in a cemetery in Stroudsburg, Pennsylvania, covered brilliantly by a profusion of wild mountain pinks and being shot over by the rifles of the National Guard honoring the Civil War dead on Decoration Day. By what inexplicable coincidence he had found a final resting-place in a town where she was later to live, she was never to discover. She is sure he must have tried, years before, to find her, when his rage and grief had ebbed. But it couldn't have been that hard to find a living child, even in the 1890s, if one really looked. Can a father forget his hapless child? Yea, he may forget.

...5

The Seventh-Day Adventist Camp Meeting in Lock Haven, Pennsylvania, must have been something to see. From all the states east of the prairies and west of the crest of the Appalachians the eager faithful came, some by train, some in wagons; whole families with furniture, dishes, bedding —all for a ten-day encampment of religious worship and renewal of faith. Lock Haven had been selected because there was a great field close enough to the residential section of town to attract converts, and because the beautiful Susquehanna River with its slow-moving current and quiet pools made possible the ritual baptism by total immersion.

The big general assembly tent was pitched in the middle of the field. Nearby was the youths' assembly tent; on the other side was the children's assembly tent. There was a dining tent where most of the campers ate one healthful meal a day at a reasonable price; there was a book tent and a reception tent. Around this central complex were pitched orderly rows of small family tents, some with floors and some without. All of the tents were white, symbolizing purity. It must have been a charming sight—all that purity laid out like fragrant fresh-washed linen on the lush summer green of the vast well-watered field.

The daily Camp Meeting schedule was rigorous. At six-thirty all the campers met in the general assembly tent for morning worship. Singing together, they sent a solemn chant of praise to God flowing across the plain, the city, and the river. It must have sounded very beautiful in the early summer mornings. After morning worship, each tent family cooked and served its own breakfast. There must have been much hurrying around; making of beds, washing of wailing children, many quick trips for water and books, much preoccupation with purely human and family concerns. Meanwhile, the ministers gathered for their business meeting before the ten-thirty sermon of the morning. All the faithful, young and old, attended the morning sermon. Almost everyone ate the main meal of the day in the dining tent, which began serving at twelve-thirty. Those who could not afford the modest fee were free to cook for themselves food that had been brought from home. At the two-thirty afternoon worship and the eight-o'clock evening meeting, the sermons were specially prepared for the public. The most appealing and skillful ministers took over at these hours, presenting the doctrines of the church: "the prophecies," "the second coming of Christ," "the mark of the beast," "the true Sabbath," and "the end of the world." In between the services, various meetings for old and young filled the day.

Harriet and the children arrived in all the happy turmoil and friendly confusion of the first Camp Meeting day. As the word spread through the encampment that a beautiful woman and her children had been "turned out of their home for the Truth's sake," everyone gathered round to admire, encourage, and help. Everything that could be done for their comfort was quickly done. Nina was thrilled by all the attention, and by the excitement of watching a special tent being put up for them in a special spot. When all was in order, she shyly edged into the first children's meeting, and by evening was walking arm in arm with little girls her own age. She went to bed happier than she had been for a long time. But happiness for Nina was not yet to be more than as a firefly fitfully shining in cupped hands, giving brief brightness without warmth.

The early-morning worship followed a set pattern. Various members of the congregation stood up to give their testimony for the Truth or to lead the others in prayer, the whole service gentled and warmed by sweet hymns. Harriet, being the prized and martyred convert, and being not unwilling to justify herself, gave her testimony early and often. She testified to the courage and faith one needs to follow God's mandate. She testified to the joy one finds when one loses the whole world to save one's immortal soul. She testified to the power of God's grace, which enabled her to remove her two innocent babes from the influence of a father who was possessed by the Devil and did the Devil's works, a number of which she itemized in detail. Nina was dizzy with shame. She loved her father and could not accept either her mother's public portrayal of him or the disloyal exposure of family affairs before strangers. She wanted to cry out that somewhere, somehow, the truth was being mutilated and torn to dress up a lie, but she sat cold and silent, shivering with fear. How did she know what was truth? Maybe her mother and these people were the truth, and her father was a lie.

One evening, at the public service, the spirit of revival was strong. Many converts, backsliders, and young children, amid tears, prayers, and songs, went forward to the mourner's bench. The organ was muted, people sang together softly, the ministers walked up and down the aisles or knelt by the mourners to talk and pray with them. Older members of the congregation led sobbing and shaken children and young people from the mourner's bench to the altar.

A kind, sweet-voiced woman put her arm around Nina. "Child," she said, "won't you come to Jesus and be saved? Jesus said, 'Suffer the little children to come unto me.'"

Nina shook her head, her eyes on the sawdust floor.

"Don't you want to be saved?" urged the voice. "Jesus is coming soon. Don't you want to be one of those who go with him to Heaven?"

Her mother bent over her. "Why don't you go with the lady and give your heart to Jesus, Nina?" she whispered. Nina looked at her mother's face, which seemed to her to be shining with holy light; she looked at the weeping congregation, and she heard the soft singing, and she took a step toward the end of the bench, the strange woman gently pulling her along. But only a step. She turned out of the woman's nudging arm and said to her mother, "I have to wait for Daddy. He is all alone."

The light dimmed in her mother's face.

"You may go back to our tent," Harriet said. As the child escaped from the hot, emotion-charged general assembly tent, she heard someone say behind her, "The spirit of God is wrestling with that child!"

On the last Sabbath before the encampment ended, baptism was celebrated. That day was the culmination of all the religious fervor, the singing, the testifying, the tears, and the exhortations of the Camp Meeting weeks. Nina was never to forget a detail of it. Two tents were pitched on the bank of the river, one for men and boys, one for women and girls. A large group of singers assembled at the water's edge. All those who had gone forward in the revival meetings were prepared for baptism. Willing hands helped them put on their baptismal robes, black for men and white for women.

Nina, Dorothy, and other children found a vantage point on a fallen tree on the bank close to the baptism pool. As the chorus sang "Washed in the Blood of the Lamb," two ministers in robes, their hands clasped before them, marched solemnly down to the river and waded out until they stood hip-deep in the water. They raised their hands for silence, and prayed. The chorus sang "Just as I Am." A man from one tent and a woman from the other went down into the river. Each one was met by one of the ministers, who wet his hands in the water and touched the brow of the convert. After both were asked and had answered questions as to their profession of faith, one minister lifted his hand and silence fell as he said, "I now baptize thee in the name of the Father, Son, and Holy Ghost." Both converts were plunged backward into the pool, to emerge sputtering and choking or with a calm joyful face, depending on their ability to hold their breath at the crucial moment. The choir sang joyful hallelujahs. The outstretched hands of brothers and sisters in the faith wrapped them in blankets and led them dripping to the tents. To Nina, it was a lovely sight. Watching the happy faces of the saved, she thought that perhaps she, too, should have gone up to the altar and should now be one of them. Then she thought that maybe someday she and her father could be baptized together. But she knew they never would be.

If I have seemed to keep us overlong at a religious Camp Meeting whose tents were folded long before any of us were born, it is because that kind of American gathering should not be totally forgotten in its detail and flavor. We know, deep and unspoken in our American hearts, that the proper place to seek for truth and beauty is out of doors. Our first settlers crossed the terrible ocean to build in our land shelters only big enough to house a family; it was out under the trees that the Thanksgiving dinner was set up, and it was the wild ones of the forest who were honored guests. The great wagon trains that moved westward joined together the just and the unjust, the weak and the brave, the craven and the strong into one efficient, indomitable organization under the scorching prairie sun and the bleak snows of the Rocky Mountains. After the era of the religious Camp Meetings, during which the Protestant egg incubated by Martin Luther hatched into a bevy of ugly ducklings scurrying in all directions, the Chautauqua Circuit took over. Culture with a capital *C* and information with political intent brought millions of our more immediate forefathers out of doors to the Chautauqua tents. Even the incomparable Sarah Bernhardt played in tent theaters on her most successful tour of the Southwest. The great American cookout has for years sent curls of aromatic smoke rising from every backyard and patio as neighbors join each other out of doors. There is, today, something deeply satisfying to the American soul that our astronauts hurl themselves into the wild blue yonder in tiny crowded spaceships and then they, and they alone, in all the universe, burst out into the open air, weightless and entranced, crying out, "I wish you were all here with me to see how beautiful this is! I don't want to go back inside."

For a few years, because of the comfortable and deadly combination of television and central air conditioning, it seemed that this great American tradition was moribund and would surely die. But in the 1960s our young people tried to save us. With their amazing instinct for tradition, they went outdoors again—our flower children to the parks

and fields, our brightest students to the barricades, our
black American young to the long, hard road from the
plantation and ghetto to the parks of Washington. The
unconquerable wanderlust of young America filled the
coves of the Greek islands, the mountain passes and super-
highways of Europe, the Peace Corps in Asia and Africa.
They were as American as Davy Crockett, Nathan Hale,
Abraham Lincoln. It was the television addicts, middle-
aged and artificially cooled, who sat inside, sour with rancor and envy, while our young moved outdoors again, looking for the good, the true, and the beautiful where, perhaps,
it can still be found. We should have more respect for our
own traditions.

...6

The last day of the Camp Meeting was, for the children, as
exciting as the first. Tents were being taken down. Everyone was packing and saying goodbye. Movement and
change and home thoughts were as vibrant in the air as the
snorting of horses and the creak of wagon wheels. It must
have been less exciting for Harriet, who now was hoisted
by her own petard. She couldn't go back to Mark. I don't
think she ever intended to go back, because she took the
books, which, in their neatly labeled boxes, were still
stacked unloaded in her wagon. Besides, she was the beautiful woman who, with her babes, had been "turned out of
her home for the Truth's sake." After playing such a role,
how could she go home again? The Lord would have to
provide. So she sat with her children on a bench by the
reception tent, watching the encampment dissolve, too
proud to ask what the church, God's instrument, would do

about her. She sat quietly, all apprehensions hidden behind a calm face and a slight asthmatic wheeze.

The Lord, and the church, did provide. A tent neighbor had already hitched Harriet's horse to her loaded wagon. As he drove it up to the reception tent, it was followed by a second wagon drawn by two prancing horses and loaded to the scuppers with supplies donated by the congregation. There was food, especially staples such as flour, rice, sugar, and home-canned vegetables. There were candles, pots and pans, including water pails and a dipper, bed linen, towels, blankets, pillows, a potbellied stove complete with flue extensions and elbow joints, pine planks for shelving, and a fine oversized tent with flooring. A young minister climbed down from the driver's seat. "These are for you and I am to drive you out to the mountains where you want to go," he said. The minister's name was Thurston Ames. They drove out of the campground with prayerful good wishes and God-bless-yous sounding in their ears. My mother remembered that Harriet was overcome with emotion and surprise.

I'll bet she really was. All of us, at least once in our lives, have had the appalling experience of stating flatly what we intend to do, fully expecting wiser, more logical, and kinder heads to reason out for us a less dangerous alternative and, with some difficulty, to persuade us out of folly. One is filled with fear and sick surprise to be cheerily ushered out into the lonely world of self-will by loving, helpful hands. Most of us have found ourselves, at least once, in the thin air of our own private self-made wilderness. Had I been Harriet, carting two trusting little children with me into an actual wilderness, I too would have been overcome by emotion—by terror. I guess she was a brave woman. Or was she so unintegrated that any role she happened to be playing was always entirely Harriet at the moment? It's difficult to know.

Thurston Ames was a jolly young man, full of health, strength, fervor, and wit. He worked hard to set up the little family so that all would be as comfortable as possible until Jesus came. He pitched the tent under a tall pine in a sheltered recess in the crags near the top of a mountain and close to a spring that people in Waterville, halfway up the mountain, had mentioned when he was seeking out an ideal site.

The spring was so extraordinary that it is still marked on the land plats of this yet underpopulated wilderness area of Pennsylvania. It was called "Sinking Spring" because the water ebbed and flowed with a tidal pattern. It was a basin about ten feet across and six feet deep. At "high tide" the water rose to the top of the basin, boiling up the white sand and shiny black flintstones, then slowly ebbed and cleared and became a placid little pool. The ceaseless movement of the water was a blessing, for it kept the spring from freezing even during the most bitter winter cold.

In the wagon there were enough pine boards not only for a floor well away from the ground, but for low walls around three sides of the tent, outside of which, and drawn somewhat underneath, the sides and back of the tent could be firmly lashed. Thurston Ames used some of the lumber to build a little outhouse, and the rest he fastened firmly as shelves along the side walls in tiers. The books that could not be accommodated on the shelves were neatly piled in their cartons up to the peak of the end wall to serve as insulation against the winter cold. He built a stone platform for the stove in the center and near the back of the tent, and spent one long, hot July afternoon keeping a roaring fire of split logs going to test the series of pipes and joints that would carry the smoke and fumes away from the tent. He stocked firewood neatly near the spring, so that if the cold came before Jesus did, one trip would provide. He boxed in fragrant hemlock boughs for aromatic beds for the family. Everyone helped him as best she could, but it was Nina to whom he turned about knotty little problems of arrangement, and it was Nina who sawed and hammered and dug and sang with him. Harriet had to be careful, for the slightest overexertion brought on agonizing attacks of asthma. Dorothy was still the baby. And it was Nina who asked him one afternoon, as he was bouncing on an arrangement of hemlock branches to test the spring of his mattress concoction, "Are you really an Adventist?"

"Of course I am," he replied. "What a funny question. Why do you ask?"

"You always seem too happy to be an Adventist."

Thurston flushed. He turned to Harriet. "Maybe I don't seem serious enough to be a minister," he said apologetically. "But what you are doing is so wonderful, and the woods are so grand, and the days are so beautiful, I feel like laughing and shouting because I'm alive. I don't think it's wrong to be happy, do you?"

Harriet's grim look softened. "No, but we must be happy in the Lord and not forget the troublous times we live in and the great burden to preach the Truth that is laid upon us." The blessing of a sense of humor is not bestowed upon us all.

Young Thurston was more silent and subdued the rest of the day. The next morning, after all had been done that he could think of to do, he hitched his young horses to his wagon. He had agreed to sell Harriet's horse for her and to send the money to the Waterville post office, so he tied the horse to the tailboard of his wagon. He kissed the children, prayed with Harriet, and left for his parish in Coudersport. For those who stayed at the tent the world must have seemed, at first, totally silent. One woman with no sense of

humor and two children with no idea of what was to happen next couldn't have been very noisy. But the birds sang,
and here and there a squirrel chattered in the forest, and
the first locusts, heralds of the thousands to come in August, tried out their rusty hymn of praise for the blessing
of the life that was to be theirs for only a moment in time.
Nina included Thurston Ames in her prayers for years.
"God bless Thurston and keep him always happy." I hope
he always was, although no one ever is, always.

...7

Somebody had to take over. The immense problem of how
to survive apart from civilization had to be solved. Harriet
wasn't the one to cope. She was again fragmented, she fell
apart, she functioned with a grim incompetence that obviously was not going to get them through the winter. Her
asthmatic attacks increased in frequency and violence every time she walked farther from the tent than the spring
or the groves of hazelnut and walnut trees nearby. I suspect
that both her asthma and her inability to plan ahead
stemmed from the same deep, blank dismay. The Lord had
always provided for Harriet, but always before through
human means; now there was nobody. Now He really had
His work cut out for Him! And Harriet was again playing
a new role, but with no audience. How could the charming
debutante, the happy wife who gave up the world for love,
the town bluestocking, the mother of many sons, the pet of
the Camp Meeting, play a new drama with only the birds
and the fat black bears and the crafty-faced, bright-eyed
wildcats for an audience? I believe she was filled with in-
capacitating dismay. After the episode of the panther, she

spent most of her time taking care of Dorothy, who was deathly afraid of leaving the tent. This is not surprising. It is not recommended as a cure for a child's fear of the forest that she be marched past the nose of a savage beast.

And so, to solve the immediate problems of survival, there was only Nina, not yet quite ten years old. She was afraid of the wild woods too, but she adopted a most unusual attitude toward her fear. As she searched the forest for nuts and berries, penetrating deeper into the unknown each day as she grew more confident of finding her way back, she said to herself, "I can no more than die, that's the worst that can happen." When she heard rustlings or creakings or snappings in the brush, she would say, "It's probably only a bunny. Anyway, the worst that can happen is that I'll be killed, then all this worry will be over. I won't have to be afraid if I'm dead."

Thus fortified with a ten-year-old's stoicism, her little heart beat less wildly and she could concentrate on finding the fresh fruits her family's diet needed, and the nuts, especially chestnuts, that she could sell in Waterville for cash to buy milk and butter at the country store. Chestnuts brought twenty cents a quart at the Waterville general store. This was good money then. She made the long trip down the mountain and the long, hard trip back twice every week because she was too small to carry a week's supply of milk in one trip.

After the episode with the panther, when the hunters stopped by to show the little family the carcass of the dead beast and to explain that it was unlikely that any of them would ever see another, because this one, they thought, must have lost his way coming down from Canada to the Rocky Mountains, Nina seized the opportunity to ask if she could get milk and butter from the Hurds, who lived, she found, only a scant three miles across the mountain instead of seven miles down. This was arranged, and when the money for the horse was finally sent, Waterville saw the child no more for the rest of the winter.

The first snow came early that year, falling softly in big, wet flakes throughout the windless night. It was the children's first sight of snow in the forest, and they were enchanted with the wonder of its whiteness and silence. Every branch and twig was bowed down under its weight. The stumps of dead, broken trees were draped as though with soft, white wool. The wilderness glowed as the rosy afternoon sun finally broke through the eastward-moving clouds.

The rest of the winter that year was mild. Very little snow fell after the first big, wet, early dump. Although it was cold, the days of bitter cold and slashing winds were infrequent. Somehow they kept warm; warm enough, at least, to avoid frostbite and chilblains. The children's shoes were still wearable, they had warm clothes, and the supplies for the winter held out. The three of them survived.

Harriet's schedule for the children's lessons was astonishing. They began at dawn and ended with dark. After morning worship, they read together one chapter of the King James version of the Bible, looking up in the dictionary all new words and analyzing sentence structure. Each child memorized three verses. The rest of the morning they read the same chapter in Latin and Greek. This was slow going at first, but for two hours every afternoon they studied Greek and Latin grammar and vocabulary. Before long the children were fluent enough to play a game that Harriet instigated. Each child looked up in the Greek and Latin dictionaries all possible meanings for one word in the chapter. The next morning, after they had tried out each separate definition, Harriet would point out the God-inspired ability of the translators of the King James Bible to choose the right meaning for the word in English. In the afternoon they studied history, mathematics, and French. This schedule was followed six days a week. On Saturday, the Sabbath, they read three chapters of the English Bible, memorized one entire chapter, and, with the aid of the church tracts, concentrated upon the religious significance of what they had read. At night, by the light of one candle, the children could read any of the textbooks or classics or novels in Harriet's library. There was no censorship. It seems curious to me that Harriet should go to such lengths to separate her children from "worldly" people and then hand them over to such authors as Shakespeare, Swift, Molière, Euripides, Catullus, and the Restoration dramatists, a far more worldly group than ever could be gathered together either in Michigan or in the Pennsylvania mountains.

So they studied and read the winter away, and one day spring came. The birds came back suddenly before it was time for birds, and the pale-blue flowers of the wild hepatica bloomed in spite of the fitful snow flurries scattered from the heavy gray skies by the cold wind. And then that day, although nothing seemed to change, the seasons changed. Something tender and gay came into the air, the branches of the trees and bushes were faintly, faintly green without reason, and the great hemlocks pushed out baby shoots, chartreuse against the somber winter needles, at the end of every separate bough.

...8

The horse money had been a gratifying amount, considering that the horse had been middle-aged and tired from hauling heavy books up hill and down dale from the flat lakelands to the Appalachians. Thurston Ames had sent

$64. Because this was more money, in the olden days, than a horse of this age should bring, I suspect that the loving-kindness in Thurston's heart had, by alchemy, turned into a few dollar bills that added themselves to whatever was paid for the horse. During the winter Nina had spent close to $15 for milk, butter, and, when the staple supplies in the tent began to run low, whatever else the Hurds could afford to sell from their own supplies. When good weather settled in, in early June, Nina stashed $30 away among the leaves of her favorite book of the moment, Guicciardini's *History of Italy,* and set out for Waterville with $19. All the way down the mountain she was uneasy and concerned about what to buy. She had tried to plan with her mother, but Harriet was not be drawn into useless discussion of practical details. "I have never seen the righteous forsaken, or his seed begging bread," she said. "Consider the lilies of the field," and, as always, "Sufficient unto the day is the evil thereof." This was frustrating for little Nina, who was concerned not about present evil but about future food.

At Waterville she enlisted the help of Dave Lovett, the owner of the general store. Between customers and incoming deliveries and his own store affairs, he discussed and advised while Nina added and subtracted flour quantities and prices to and from the quantities and prices of rice, sugar, lentils, shelled corn, and Mrs. Lovett's home-canned vegetables. Finally, after agonizing reappraisals, she was ready with her list. Mr. Lovett, with real appreciation for her logic and arithmetic, approved her choices and, because there was at the moment only one other customer in the store, who was busy with his own list, sat down at the counter with her to discuss the problem of getting the supplies up the mountain to the tent. It was a knotty problem. Mr. Lovett was a "city" man; he lived in the village, did no farming, and had no horse or wagon. Nina had no money for drayage. Her hidden $30 was stored away against the coming of the next winter. It might not last, but it was all the money there was, unless money, like manna, came from parts unknown.

The young farmer puzzling over his own supplies was named Jake Burton. He lived in a cabin across the crest of the mountain past the tent, and his life was hard. Although he was only in his early thirties, he had six children. His wife was a shrew and a slattern and his children were wild, undisciplined, and unloving. He scratched a sort of living out of his own little rocky fields and hired himself out to more affluent farmers for cash. He had become surly. He seldom spoke, never fraternized, and looked upon other people's problems with the stony, cruel indifference of the overburdened.

All of a sudden Jake Burton, who, because he couldn't help it, had been listening to the discussion between the child and the man, turned and came to the counter. "I'll take the kid's gear up the mountain for her," he said. Nina glowed with gratification.

"That's wonderful!" she exclaimed, and turned to Mr. Lovett, who sat with such a look of open-mouthed surprise that she stopped short. Years later she told me that Mr. Lovett looked to her at that moment as though he were seeing the angel Gabriel. Since she was young and open-hearted, she turned back to Jake and said, "You must be the angel Gabriel!" Both of the men stared open-mouthed at the child. Perhaps neither of them knew who the angel Gabriel was, or perhaps the introduction of a heavenly being into the general store of Waterville, Pennsylvania, was shocking, but both of them stared at her with such blank incomprehension that the child was momentarily abashed.

It is a curious thing that evil and panic and blood lust

spread in a mob as the Black Death spread through medie-
val cities, but kindliness spreads only from person to person, tentatively and modestly. It doesn't seem fair to goodness that evil is so much more contagious. Jake Burton was
infected either by the assurance in the child's voice that
what had to be done could somehow be done or by the
patience and concern of Mr. Lovett. At any rate, he caught
kindness. He explained that he had a full load of his own
supplies to take up the mountain that day, but that "the
kid" could ride up with him in the wagon with what she
could carry on her lap, and the next week, when he returned to the Waterville foundry to pick up a plow that was
being repaired, he would haul her gear to the tent. "As in
water face answereth to face, so the heart of man to man."
Given a start, that is, by some invisible prod, and not always then.

Nina used the trip back with Jake Burton to find out
from him all he knew about food that could be found in the
forest before the season of berries and nuts arrived. She
knew that the small bundle of supplies on her lap, added
to the dregs of the winter's store, would not last the week
unless she could supplement them with the wild products
of the mountain. He told her about dandelion greens; he
stopped the wagon to show her how to find mushrooms and
how to tell the poisonous ones from the good. He pointed
out a trail into the woods that eventually would lead to a
burned-out wilderness of dead trees where a strange, early-
ripening berry, long and thin like a finger, could already be
found. She was cheerful and serene when they parted, sure
she could manage to feed the three of them until Jake Burton came again.

It wasn't easy. They had found, late in the winter, that
corn parched and pounded to a fine meal and then cooked
made a delicious mush. They had some flour for bread,

some brown rice, some butter and milk, a little sugar and a little salt. Harriet used salt sparingly, lest it inflame the baser passions.

The morning after her trip Nina went out at dawn to find mushrooms. She was far up a strange trail, carefully choosing good mushrooms from bad, when she heard twigs snapping behind her as birds flew up with sharp twitterings. A large black bear emerged from the woods from the right of the path about a hundred yards away. The bear stood for a moment, then began slowly moving toward her. She turned away and flew down the path, the skin on her back tightening in anticipation of a blow of the bear's paw. At the end of the trail, in a clearing, was a mountaineer's cabin. She raced into the open door, slammed it shut, and with bursting lungs leaned against it, gasping. The woman inside sprang up and went to the window. Nothing was in view. Turning, she asked, "What was after you? There ain't nothing."

"A bear! A big bear!" Nina gasped, going to the window. Just then the bear ambled out into the clearing, turned by the edge of the woods, and went down the path toward the spring.

"He warn't after ye. He could've ketched ye any time. He was just goin' your way," said the woman. "Bars only git after people when they is cornered or got young uns. He's just tryin' to get fed up good atter bein' holed up all winter. Set and rest, child. You're plum done up. You're one of them kids that live in the tent, ain't ye?"

"Yes, I am. I think I lost my faith for a little while," Nina said.

"Lost what?" asked the woman, puzzled.

"My faith. You know. God said nothing can harm anyone who is his child, but I forgot when the bear came at me. I should have been praying unceasingly," she said.

"Who teached you that?" asked the woman. "Your ma?"
"Yes," the child replied gravely. "She reads it in the Bible."

After thanking the woman, she went home. She didn't mention the bear to her mother and sister. The mushrooms were delicious and not a poison one among them.

A week later, when Jake Burton still had not come, Nina set out to find the forest of dead trees in order to pick the berries he had called "timber berries." After a long hike along the faint trail made by animals in search of food, she arrived. It was awesome. Acres of once giant trees of pine, chestnut, oak, and hemlock stood stark and barkless, grayish-white, with broken limbs sticking up toward Heaven. As if to emphasize the barren loneliness, a few crows flew with raucous caws, lighting on the leafless arms and stubs of the spectral trees; black, shining, aggressive crows as large as ravens and unintimidated by desolation. The undergrowth of thick chestnut and oak shoots, mixed with the timber-berry bushes, was almost impassable. The day was warm and windless and, except for the intermittent harsh cry of the crows, entirely silent. Nina plunged into the underbrush, dropping timber berries into her ten-quart pail as she pushed and scratched her way through. She talked aloud to herself. She always did in times of uncertainty and danger. Even when she was old, she would suddenly begin to talk to herself, fortifying herself against the panic aroused by awareness of loss of health, vigor, and usefulness. "I'll bet the ghosts of these old trees are in the briars clustered around them," she said. "But they're not terrible ghosts. They're only little ghosts, cross and scratchy. I guess I'd be cross, too, if I had once been an ancient, beautiful tree."

After her bucket was full, she climbed upon a rotting log, putting the bucket carefully on a wide, flat place between two knots of wood. She had turned so many ways picking berries that she was unsure of the direction from which she had entered the dead forest. She spotted the opening of the faint trail and started to slide down from the log when she heard a shrill, thin, ominous rattle that whirred and burred until the terrible sound seemed to fill all the air. Down below, among the rocks that held the log high off the ground, was coiled a seething mass of yellow and black flesh, a flat, bright, burnished head held high, a red tongue flickering and darting at her. "It's the Devil himself," she cried aloud as she threw herself backward over the other side of the log just as the snake struck. He missed her by inches and fell with a dull, flat thud into the rocks below where she had fallen. She sprang up as the rattler, with incredible rapidity, was already recoiling his heavy body, and scrambled along the rocks to a safe distance. From there she looked back at her berries, which were needed so badly at home. She hesitated, debating if she should go back. It is a terrible thing to have to learn the ways of wild creatures by trial and error and by judgment unacquainted with the essential nature of the enemy. Mountain children learned from others. Nina didn't know what to do. Almost immediately the air was again filled with the shrill menacing rattle, which is as deadly to the spirit as the venom is to the blood. The child turned and ran, clawing and pushing her way through the underbrush deeper and deeper into the dead forest until she was completely lost.

When darkness came she was still scrambling through the underbrush, but she could see the end of the burned-over ground and the beginning of the open forest. Darkness came early as the sky clouded over and the low, intermittent thunder of an approaching storm grumbled. Crows flapped slowly and dismally ahead of her. Within the edge of the forest the darkness became so thick and the child was so exhausted that she had to stop. She sank down to the ground, her back snuggled up against a large tree. "At least nothing can get me from behind," she said. Worn out by fear and exertion, she slept.

The storm was slow in coming, but finally the thick spat-spat of the rain on the leaves and the chill drops on her face awoke her. Before long, the full force of the storm broke over the forest and the child was drenched. She huddled against the tree trunk. As the great claps of thunder began to pass on, she thought she heard a dog barking. Cupping her hands, she shouted into the night. Now she was almost sure she heard a dog barking, nearer. Maybe it's wolves, she thought, and for a while could hear nothing but her own pounding heart. But the dog barked again, still nearer. "No, it's a dog. Thank God, it's a dog. Here, Shep! Here, Shep!" she called.

"Oh, dog, take me out!" she sobbed as a big, wet shepherd dog, after barking and smelling around her, finally licked her hands and face as she huddled close to the tree. If ever there is a time to cry, it is in a night of sorrow when the muzzle of a dog sniffles, and the warm, wet tongue caresses a friend. Clinging to the dog, she set out into the night and the rain and, after a while, arrived at a cabin. Nothing stirred at the dog's short, sharp barks, so the child pounded on the door.

"Who's that?" a rough male voice called.

"Please open the door and let me in," cried the child. There was a pause and the scratch of matches. An old man, lamp in hand, opened the door.

"My God! Where did you come from?" he said as the child staggered in, still clinging to the dog, and sank into a wet, bedraggled heap on the dry dirt floor.

The farmer's name was Wally Zinskinsky, "Old Wally." He took off the child's sodden dress and wrapped her in a dirty horse blanket. He forced a teaspoon of moonshine whiskey between her teeth. As Nina sputtered and choked she looked at the hairy old man. Oh! I'm in an ape's den, she thought in despair.

"Don't be afraid," he said gruffly. "Go to sleep—tell me in the morning." The dog licked her face. I guess I'm safe, she thought, and sank into a dreamless sleep.

...9

Although Nina didn't know it, a new era in her life began the next morning. When she stumbled into the Zinskinskys' cabin, drained of strength and courage, she stumbled into an end to the lonely responsibility of keeping three people alive. From now on, a new road to food and money and human contact would be open to her.

The rhythmic fall of an axe near the window awakened her. Sun was streaming in through the open door. Her clothes were folded and dry on a nearby stool. A tall, untidy girl of sixteen and a thirteen-year-old boy stood looking at her.

"How be ye?" asked the girl.

"What's your name?" asked the boy.

"My name's Nina Mae Case. What's yours?"

"Mine's Booby and hern is Mary," answered the boy. "How old are ye?"

"I'm ten, going on eleven," Nina answered. "Where's your mother?"

Mary answered, "She ain't here now. She runned away again."

"Ran away? Oh, how awful! Can't you find her?"

"Pa don't want us to. We don't look for her no more. She

used to run off and git drunk, but she always come back
when she sobered. Last fall, Pa beat her good to learn her
better, and Ma went off. We hear about her sometimes from
lumbermen and barkmen, but she don't come home no
more." Mary flushed. Booby turned and walked out of the
cabin.

While Mary started breakfast, Nina dressed and went
out to the woodpile. Old Wally didn't look so terrible in the
new-washed morning world.

"Well," he said, leaning on his axe, "who be ye, and how
come ye here in a night storm?"

"I'm Nina Case, and my mother and my sister and I live
in a tent over on Smokey Hill." She told him what had
happened the day before. The old man chuckled grimly.

"You was right to run from a rattler," he said. "Your
mom'll be worrit about ye and it's nigh eight miles to
Smokey Hill."

"Mother won't worry," the child said. "She'll think I
must have gone on to Waterville to sell part of the berries.
She put me in God's care, so she won't worry."

The old man looked at her strangely. "What do ye mean,
'in God's care'?" he asked.

"Why, she asks God to take care of me and then she
doesn't have to worry."

"Then she won't be cryin' and huntin' for you this morning?"

"No, why should she? No, indeed. She and Dorothy will
sing 'Lord in the Morning' and ask Him to bring me home
safely with something to eat today." Nina sighed. "And
that old rattler got my berries."

Old Wally shook his head. "Your mother must be fey, as
I heerd tell."

Nina was indignant. "My mother's wonderful!"

"Thar, thar, course she's wonderful. Tell me, how do ye
eat? Where do ye get food?"

"God sees we have enough," Nina assured him. "We've never been a whole day without food. It looked pretty much like it two days ago. Mother had one of her bad spells with asthma, and I couldn't go into the woods for food. We had corn cakes for breakfast and used the last we had. My little sister asked, 'Now what will we have for dinner?' Mother said, 'The Lord will provide. Let's ask Him.' So while we prayed, we heard a man say, 'Whoa,' at the end of our path on the road. We walked down and he called to us to find out where he was. He was afraid he'd taken the wrong turn to go by the short cut to Coudersport to sell a whole wagonload of wintered potatoes. He sure had taken the wrong turn! Wasn't it wonderful that he came our way? He sold Mother two bushels of potatoes for her watch and chain. We had a wonderful dinner of potatoes baked in the ashes of our stove. I guess we'll have to eat potatoes again today, unless Mr. Burton comes."

Old Wally was as startled as Mr. Lovett had been to hear that Jake Burton would do any favors for anyone. "Ye musta witched him," he said. Nina laughed. She said she should start home.

Not to be outdone by Jake Burton, Old Wally bridled his horse and rode Nina two-thirds of the way home. He claimed he had to go to arrange for Injun Jake Dutter, a half-breed who lived with his mother not far from Smokey Hill, to bug potatoes the next day. And maybe he did have to go. But kindness *is* contagious, from person to person. On the way, Nina arranged to hire herself out for potato-bugging in exchange for twenty-five cents a day and findings, which would include lunch and whatever milk, vegetables, meal, and supplies Old Wally had extra, and as much as he would think her work would be worth.

Harriet was appalled at the idea of Nina's working for Old Wally.

"But you are not of this world, and you mustn't associate

with those who are reserved for the second death," she argued. "No, I cannot let you."

"But Mother, we are in this world, and until Jesus comes, we have to eat. Even Jesus ate with publicans and sinners," Nina replied.

"So He did," said Harriet, startled. "Well, we'll pray about it."

The upshot of the prayers was that Nina could walk the eight miles back and forth every day, work all day in the summer sun, and bring home sustenance. The Lord will provide. Consider the lilies of the field. I would say to myself, "Poor child!" except that she was happy. She didn't have to worry any more. Winter would not find her unprepared.

The work was hard at first. She and Old Wally and Injun Jake bugged potato hills for several days. Each worker had a short stick and a pail partly filled with kerosene. Bending down to the potato hill, Nina put her pail under the leaves and brushed sharply against the stalks, shaking the potato bugs off into the pail. She then picked off the leaves that had yellow eggs on them and put them also into the kerosene. The sun was hot and the kerosene smell was strong. The first day, as they trudged back to the cabin for the noon meal, Nina was glad to leave the smothering fumes behind her with her pail. But she was appalled to sit down to the dinner Mary had prepared. I guess Mother's right, she thought. I guess we aren't the same kind of people. Dinner consisted of boiled potatoes, fried side pork, sour black bread, and coffee. According to her religion, Nina could not eat pork, and coffee was Satan's brew, so all she could eat were potatoes and sour bread. Old Wally was amazed and Mary was offended.

"Seems like your religion is for rich folks," she said. "Usuns eat what we can git and thank God for it."

Nina was thoughtful the rest of the afternoon. It would be nice, she thought, to just eat and sleep and live without the fear that Jesus would suddenly come and make snap judgments on the basis of one day's transgressions.

But as summer drew on and Nina worked six days a week, every day but Saturday, the Sabbath, the work was often fun and sweet-smelling. She raked the hay and helped pitch it into the wagon, and she helped stow it away in the barn. She dug potatoes, husked corn, learned to milk. Every week brought something new, and every day brought twenty-five cents and all the food she could carry home. Old Wally was a good man.

...10

The second winter was uneventful. In many ways it was more pleasant than the first, the way anything is after routine and know-how have been established. The intense program of study was more interesting for them all. By then the children were reasonably fluent in Greek and Latin, and in the afternoon they read plays and poems and essays in the original language. Harriet added geography and Eastern religions to the course of study. The children had developed physically and mentally, and had grown accustomed to living vicariously in books and imagination.

They also had grown out of their shoes. Nina's shoes were worn out, and her dresses were almost in shreds from her work in the fields and her wandering in the forest. Dorothy could still wear her shoes with the toes cut out, but Nina was shoeless. To go to the spring for water, or to the pheasant traps that Booby had taught her to make, or to the woodpile, she wrapped burlap bags around her feet and tied them around her ankles. Nina was always merry whenever there was a moment when she could be, and as she clowned with her oversized burlap-wrapped feet, prancing like a puss-in-boots, even Harriet and Dorothy had to laugh. It couldn't have been easy to amuse those two.

Winter came to an end, as winters always do, and in early May Nina set out for Old Wally's farm to begin work. Even before she entered the cabin she could hear Booby calling wildly for his mother. Old Wally and Mary were in despair. Booby had been "taken" with a mysterious fever a week before, which had risen each day until the boy was delirious, barely alive in a nightmare of constantly losing and finding and losing his mother. Nina was frightened. "My mother could help him, she knows what to do for fever," she told Wally. "But you'll have to let Mary drive over for her. She can't walk this far."

Harriet and Dorothy came back with Mary in the wagon. It was the first time Harriet had left the tent since she came to the mountains. She brought with her the only medicines she had, niter and castor oil, and poured a dose of each down the raving child's throat. She wrapped him in a wet sheet and alternately dripped ice-cold water over him and spooned herb tea into his mouth. The high fever began to abate, and in little more than an hour the desperately sick child was conscious and able to take more liquid into his dehydrated body. Harriet told Wally to send for the boy's mother. "I'm afraid she will never see him alive unless she comes soon." Wally stood looking stubborn. "Don't delay," Harriet urged. "If he sees her, it may save his life."

Wally turned to Mary. "Go git Kathy," he said. "Tell her Booby's adyin' and wants her."

Nina begged, "Oh, Mother, may I go with her? Maybe I can help persuade her to come." Harriet agreed that she could go.

"Don't worry ifen we don't git back tonight," Mary warned. "If she ain't in Waterville, she maybe is up Pine Creek. It'll take some lookin'."

"Hurry!" said Harriet. "This boy is sick unto death."

The girls raced down the mountain in record time and asked for Kathy at the hotel. Yes, Kathy had been there Saturday night, but no one knew where she was staying. They went to the general store. Mr. Lovett knew. "Yes, she was in here yesterday," he said. "She lives up on the Gooseberry with Old Man Yetter, if they ever got there from here. Both of them were so drunk they had to hold each other up when they staggered up the road. What do you want with Kathy?"

"Her boy is dying. We've got to find her. How do we find Old Man Yetter's place?" asked Nina.

"You can't miss it. There are only two cabins on Gooseberry Mountain and his is the first one." He led them outside and pointed to an opening in the hills. "It's four or five miles up that road. You kids have any dinner?" The girls shook their heads. "Well, you can't walk up that steep road on an empty stomach. Come back in and I'll fix you a lunch."

"We ain't got no money," muttered Mary, backing down the steps.

"Don't need none," replied Mr. Lovett, hurriedly putting crackers, cheese, dried beef, and apples into a sack. Nina thanked him and offered to bring him chestnuts later to pay for the food. "No you won't," he said. "Pity if I can't help a sick boy by giving you a little lunch. Get along or you'll be caught by the dark in the woods."

The girls climbed steadily for some time and then, exhausted by the steep, rocky road, sat down by a little run of water to eat. The view over the budding green valley was wonderful. "It just rests me to look at that stream wandering there down in the valley," Nina said.

"It don't rest me none," said Mary. "If we don't find Mom at Yetter's, I'm going back. She probably won't come anyway."

"Yes, she will. No one would refuse to go to a dying person," Nina said confidently.

"You don't know my mom. If she says she won't, then she won't."

They came, finally, to the cabin. A dog barked. A woman put her head out of an upstairs window. My mother remembered that the woman had beautiful white curls springing crisply above a tanned handsome face slightly raddled by an obvious hangover. "That's Mom!" exclaimed Mary. They knocked and a man opened the door.

"What do you want?"

"We want Kathy."

"She ain't here."

"Oh, yes, she is, Mr. Yetter," Nina said. "We saw her stick her head out of the window. Come on down, Kathy," she called. "Come down! Booby is dying and he wants you. My mother says you must come. His blood will be on your hands if you don't."

With a clatter of feet on the stairs, Kathy came down. She was trembling. "What blood? What blood? My God, my head's killin' me! What's this about Booby and blood?"

Kathy left with the girls, but part way down the mountain they met a man staggering, as my mother said, under a load of drink. His name was Sam. He and Kathy were old-time drinking friends, and when Sam pulled a bottle of moonshine whiskey out of his pocket, they sat down on a rock. Sam took a swig and passed the bottle to Kathy, who took a long pull.

Mary said, "Come on, Nina, we're done for. She won't come now."

Kathy passed the bottle back and Sam motioned with it

to the girls. "Come on, kids, take a little drink, do you good. Come on, take it, take it," holding the bottle out to Nina. She walked up to him, took the bottle, and threw it over the cliff. It struck and rolled and crashed down through the brush and into the rocks below, and all was still. Sam roared with shock and dismay. Kathy, fortified by her drink, laughed, got up, and left with the children while Sam was still trying to get to his feet. Stronger now, Kathy set such a fast pace that the girls had to run to keep up with her.

They were climbing Helmsville Mountain along Pine-bottom Run when darkness closed in. Only the ribbon of starshine over the narrow road kept them on their way. Kathy had to slow her pace as the girls stumbled over roots and stones. "We'll cut up Rattlesnake Run," she said.

"Oh, no, Mom!" Mary was frightened. "Pop says never to go that way no more. There's some men living in the Fry shanty and Pop thinks they's escaped convicts."

Kathy grunted. "Whoever's thar can't be no worse than I seen already. Come on. We'll git a lantern thar, or a torch. Come on! Come on!" as the girls hung back.

It was so dark on the overgrown path that they could not see each other. Kathy broke off a long stick and the girls, stumbling and numb from exhaustion, hung on to the stick. "I can walk this path," Kathy said, "if it's darker 'n hell. Many's the time I done it."

There was a light in the Fry cabin. Kathy rapped on the door with a stick. The light went out, the back door squeaked, and Kathy yelled, "Hey! Open up this door, you polecats, or I'll bust it in." Silence.

"Who the hell are you?" said a voice behind them.

"We need a lantern and something to eat," Kathy said.

"We ain't got no lantern, and we don't hold with strangers hangin' around. Git goin'!"

By this time three other men, each coming from a different part of the woods, joined the first. Someone struck a match and held it to Kathy's face. "Well! If it ain't Kathy!" he exclaimed. "Come on in. But what about them kids?"

"They're all right," Kathy assured the men. "They won't talk. One's mine and this 'n," pointing to Nina, "is so done out she don't know her ass from a hole in the ground."

Inside the cabin, when her eyes had adjusted to the relit kerosene lamps, Nina looked around in amazement. Exactly in the middle of the only room was a huge black machine. Underneath, it had a kind of giant treadle, and it had a big flat round top. Could it be a sewing machine? Across one wall was a long work table littered with tools and rolls of heavy paper. Kathy motioned the two girls to one of the bunks. They sat down and within minutes both of them were fast asleep.

Kathy woke them two hours later. As they struggled to their feet, Nina saw one of the men give Kathy a handful of money. "Take it to Ed King," he said. "But don't spend none until he gives 'em the once-over. If he wants some, come back and tell us when and where to deliver."

Outside the cabin, one of the men was splitting a pine knot into long slivers until he had two bunches. He lit the first sliver and, as it began to burn, added one sliver after another and handed them to Kathy as a torch. The second bundle he divided between the two children to carry as spares. "This'll hold you with light till you git thar. You can stick the burned ones in the ground to put 'em out when they's burned up."

Kathy laughed and thwacked the bearded man on the back. "Boy," she said, "I made torches 'fore ye was borned!" All the men laughed. Mother remembered that she was too dazed with weariness to laugh with them. Kathy and her retinue marched off into the night.

It was past three o'clock in the morning when they stumbled into Old Wally's lane. Kathy extinguished the torches and steered Mary and Nina toward the barn.

"Go sleep in the hay. I'll tell 'em where ye be," she said, and strode into the house.

The noon sun was high when the girls awoke. Nina was sore in every muscle. After a sedentary winter of reading, translating, quoting, and discussing, eighteen hours of rigorous hiking made themselves felt. She hobbled into the house with Mary.

"Where's Ma?" Mary asked Harriet.

"She's gone. She left an hour ago. Booby is better. His temperature is down and he's sleeping like a baby." Harriet looked at Mary and said, with wonderment, "Your mother is a remarkable woman."

Kathy was indeed remarkable. Born and bred to be the wife of a mountain farmer—a life of boredom, drudgery, abuse, and disrespect—she broke away at terrible cost; to her husband, Old Wally, who was a good man, but a wife-beater in the days when beating a wife was normal relief from frustration; to her children, who loved her and forgave her continually in return for a few motherly crumbs; and to herself. I don't doubt that she died early from alcoholic poisoning or from falling off a mountain cliff. But she was life-loving and an Amazon. She escaped the fate of other ignorant mountain wives, which was an equally early death from overwork and hopelessness. And where could she escape to, illiterate, untrained, and penniless? Lumbermen, barkmen, counterfeiters liked her, and if they didn't treat her as a lady, they treated her as a person, which is sometimes the most important thing in the world.

Booby's recovery was, for Harriet, the beginning of a brief but true renaissance. I can safely judge that this was so because my mother once said that after Booby was saved from death, Harriet slowly became the capable and vigorous woman she had been before her baby died. The story of her success in saving Booby spread over the scattered mountain community. Wagons began arriving at the tent more and more frequently to take "Hattie," as they called her to her indignation, to the bed of someone in fever and pain, in childbirth, or with uncontrolled bleeding from accidents with axes or falling rocks. She did well. She was a brilliant woman. She had read widely. Her church's emphasis on health and herbal medicine gave her tools to work with, and gave her confidence. She was both inventive and cautious. As her modest fame grew, her asthma waned. As she entered more and more into her Florence Nightingale role, she even began to robe herself in a special, freshly laundered nurselike uniform when she was sent for. She began to worry less about who was "reserved for the second death" and, with surprising success, saved from the first death those in dire distress and danger. She left religious tracts with her patients, in hope of also saving souls, but, unfortunately, most of her patients were unable to read.

It was during this period that Nina's determination to be a doctor was formed. She couldn't have had many opportunities, until then, to admire her mother objectively. Children seldom do. The poor little things are trapped in the dreadful world of childhood where they must love their mothers and depend upon them because there is, actually and literally, nothing else to do. Mother has to be right because she is indispensable. But Nina had had the unique experience of being, from the age of nine, the sole means of physical support for her indispensable mother. And then suddenly, when Nina was eleven, going on twelve, her mother entered Nina's world. In one soft sweet flowering gentle spring day, Harriet became to her child a partner in survival and a source of public pride. It is little wonder that this transient role that Harriet was playing crystallized into an adamantine resolve for a child who had been so hard beset, so frightened, and who was, by nature, so single-minded as to walk, singing hymns, straight past panthers. Nina decided she would become a doctor.

One Sunday, part of the chapter she had memorized for her Sunday-morning lesson haunted her mind all afternoon. "Verily I say unto you, if ye have faith as a grain of mustard seed, ye shall say unto this mountain, Remove hence to yonder place; and it shall remove; and nothing shall be impossible unto you." All afternoon the phrase "and nothing shall be impossible unto you" kept running through her mind.

"Mother, how big is a mustard seed?" she asked that evening.

"Why," Harriet answered, "it is a tiny little seed."

"How little? Show me," Nina persisted.

Harriet looked around for something small as a mustard seed. She finally separated one grain of sugar from the sugar bowl.

"About this size, only round," she said.

"That *is* a little seed," Nina declared. "Anybody ought to be able to grow that much faith. I'm going to start in right now and have faith. What exactly does it mean, 'have faith as a grain of mustard seed'?"

"Well," Harriet responded, "do you remember the first chapter in the Bible when God created the heavens and the earth? He spoke and it was. If we had some of that power, even as small a piece as a mustard seed, nothing would be impossible. That is faith."

"I want to go to school, and I want to be a doctor when I grow up," Nina announced, with shining eyes. "I'm starting today to have faith that this will come to pass."

Harriet was appalled. "Women can't be doctors. Only men are allowed to go to medical school. For a woman, there isn't the ghost of a chance. Besides, surely Jesus will come before you're old enough. Have faith in something sensible."

Look who was talking!

Dismayed, Nina wandered out of the tent and down to the Sinking Spring. The moonlight glinted on the water that was boiling up so mysteriously from deep in the earth. And nothing shall be impossible unto you, she thought. I'll just start having faith, anyway, that I'll be a doctor. And I'll add an extra mustard seed of faith that Jesus won't come before I *am* a doctor. Because of my mustard seed, the Lord will have to wait.

We know now, from where we stand, that He waited.

...11

June was a lovely month, misty with recurring pearly fogs that spiraled up from the lowlands, obscuring in soft gray swirls all the harshness of the forests; fogs that shimmered creamy gold in the late-morning sun before spiraling into nothingness above the fresh green leaves. Wagons clanked almost daily to the tent for Harriet and Dorothy. Both of them bloomed from their new association with the mountain folks. Every morning except the Sabbath Nina went to work with Old Wally, Injun Jake, and Booby. There was plenty of food in the tent, and the little family had much to relate to each other in the lingering summer evenings. All was well. July came in hot, but with brisk winds that ripened the hay in the modest scattered meadows. All was well until little Nina was bitten by a rattlesnake.

Old Wally, Injun Jake, Booby, and Nina had just returned from one of Mary's noontime dinners. Nina was
carefully picking her way across the brush and rocks piled
along the wagon trail at the edge of the big meadow when
all at once the ominous rattle she had heard once before
began to shrill and rose to a high, piercing whine.

"Rattlesnake!" she cried aloud.

She couldn't see the snake. She put her foot out into the
clearest space to step back into the road when the snake
struck, almost knocking her over. She screamed and sprang
out into the road, dragging the snake with her until the
flesh tore from the side of her foot and the rattler slid away
into the rocks. Scream after terrified scream brought Old
Wally running across the field.

"Sit down! Sit down right in the road," he shouted.

Nina sank down holding her foot, still screaming. As he
ran Old Wally pulled out his pocket knife, and when he
reached her he pulled up her foot between his legs as
though to shoe a horse. He sucked the wound strongly,
spitting out the blood and venom over and over again.
Then he cut out the wound, wide and deep, helping it to
bleed freely. Nina fainted. When the wound stopped bleeding he packed it with tobacco from his pouch, picked up the
unconscious child, and carried her to the barn, where Jake
and Booby were already harnessing the horses to the
wagon. They drove wildly over the rutted mountain trails
to the tent. Harriet undressed the child and got her into
bed. She commended Old Wally for his bloodletting but
expressed grave concern about the use of the tobacco.

"Tobacco is an ugly weed. It was the Devil who sowed
the seed," she said.

"Well," said Old Wally, "it was all I had to do with, and
it shore is turnin' green, ain't it?"

Whether because of the abundant bleeding, the tobacco

greening, or the grace of God, the child, after a week of pain and crisis, began to recover.

One result of the snakebite from which she was never to recover was the effect of bright sunlight on her eyes. In the first few weeks, any strong light, no matter how indirect, caused nausea and severe pain behind her eyes. Gradually, however, she was able to go out on sunny days if she wore a sunbonnet. In those times sunbonnets in the country and hats in town were commonplace. Years later she was to become famous for her beautiful hats, intricately decorated creations that she wore with her crisp white doctor's coat as she made the rounds of her patients in the hospital or in their homes. When the American Medical Association feted her on her fiftieth year of medical practice, making her Pennsylvania's Woman of the Year, the association presented her not only with a plaque, but also with a hat covered with masses of pale pink roses to rest lightly on her lovely white hair. Fifty years before, when she began her medical practice, the men doctors, affronted at the idea that a woman should be allowed to practice medicine, were mollified whn Dr. Nina wore a new creation of a hat to each monthly meeting of the county medical society; now their sons and grandsons were amused and softened, made courtly and condescending by what they considered a charming feminine foible in a lady doctor much older and wiser than they. They could not see the rattlesnake among the roses.

The most important result of the snakebite was that the three of them in the tent had to leave the mountain. They could not weather another winter without Nina to provide. The gifts of food that Harriet received in payment for her Florence Nightingale act, along with the nuts and berries and fruits that kindly neighbors, almost as poor as our little family, would leave at the end of the tent lane for "the young 'un," would provide only until the cold weather threatened, with its inexorable demand that there be a winter's supply of staples bought, paid for, and delivered to the tent. Harriet's asthma, which had returned when Nina was stricken, was complicated by the onset of arthritis in her neck and knees and fingers.

Harriet prayed for guidance all during July and early August. I would bet she also prayed that the Lord would come now, now, now, so that the need to act would be canceled. But by mid-August, when nothing had changed, she wrote to her aunt in the Pennsylvania town not so very far away to ask for house room for the winter. In late August, when Nina was well enough to go into Waterville for the mail, the reply came that the aunt had died some years before, and the uncle felt no call to take in those who were not his own blood kin. Then Harriet rewrote her plea both to the church elders and to her aunt in Philadelphia, the other heir of her parents' estate.

...12

September was beautiful. It almost seemed as though the whole forest, the whole summer, were saying, "Look at me! See how gentle, how green, how pretty I am! Where will you ever again find such a place, so beautiful and so benign?" No early frost began the coloring of the leaves. Only the country-butter-yellow goldenrod and the bright light blue of the flowering thistles and the dark, strong red of the berry bushes, whose color change does not depend on frost, confirmed the cold to come. All else was sunshine and lusty green, with birds chirping and collecting for flight and not yet going; an occasional dark bear in a green tree gorging on amber honey; and the squirrels, nature's most perfect rodents, cynically gathering their nuts with incessant chatterings and clatterings, knowing that winter and famine and deprivation lurk behind the façade of unnatural benevolence.

One green-gold late-September morning, Nina, sunbonneted, was early in the woods looking for food. As she walked, thoughts flickered in her mind and Bible verses came and went. This is not strange, considering the exposure she had had to the Bible. All of a sudden she said aloud, "Do with your might what your hands find to do, and the Lord will make room for you." She was pleased. She knew she was joining two separate verses from two disparate parts of the Old Testament. She knew she was misquoting each one of them. But at that moment in the September forest, this concise verbal statement of basic philosophy was profoundly pleasing.

Do you suppose that each of us, in puberty, already carries within himself the person he will be for the next sixty years? Is one's whole life form contained in one's temperament, to be sharpened and augmented by experience, education, and age, but never to be changed basically by any of these? Does the mating of the genes of two adults produce a child able to look at reality with only a single eye and to cope with the world in only one predestined, esoteric way? For Nina, who was to live eighty more years, work was to be the reality, the key to unlock a place that was to be her own in the crowded, strange, and indiscriminatory world.

On that green-gold September day, Nina, pleased with her philosophy, started a game, just as any child would do. Stretching her arms out wide, eyes closed, she swiveled left to right, right to left in as wide an arc as she could reach. At a given mystic moment, she stopped, opened her eyes, and sighted along her left arm. Nothing but forest and dappled sunlight. But along the axis of her right arm, far back off the trail, sat a red squirrel. Feeling himself watched, he flicked around and dived into a hollow log almost covered by brambles. By the time Nina reached the log, it was squirrelless but full of hundreds of chestnuts.

"Well, hands," she rejoiced aloud, "you found something sure enough!"

She searched through the brambles until she found a long stick with a stump of a branch near the end making a hook, and using it as a rake, she had more than a bushel of nuts piled on the ground. Gathering up her long, ragged skirt, she filled it with as many as it would hold and started back to the tent. "Here I come," she said, "just like Ruth with wheat in her dress!" After two more trips, she had all the chestnuts safely stored in gunnysacks to be taken to Waterville.

"You know, Mother," she said as they were eating a lunch of roasted chestnuts, dandelion greens, and buttermilk, "my hands found these nuts."

"What on earth do you mean, your hands found them?" asked Harriet impatiently.

"Well, I was thinking of that Bible verse, 'Whatsoever thy hand findeth to do, do it with thy might,' and I stretched out my hands and told them to get busy. My hands found a squirrel near an old hollow log, and there were all the nuts."

"I guess the Lord sent food to us this way," said Harriet, "instead of by ravens, as he did to Elijah." She didn't notice how pale and tired and hot her eleven-year-old daughter was, exhausted by being God's raven.

A few days later, Nina pulled and dragged two gunnysacks full of chestnuts down the mountain to the Waterville general store, taking care to keep to the high, grassy crown of the wagon road and to ease the sacks over the outcroppings of sharp flintstone and limestone that ridged the road at random spots. She had tied a two-gallon covered milk pail around her waist with a rope, and she eased herself and her burden down the mountain with rustlings and clinks and clanks.

With the money Dave Lovett gave her for the nuts, she ate a lunch of bread and cheese and milk. With flour, sugar, and salt in a gunnysack in one hand and her pail full of fresh milk, with a roll of country butter floating in it, in the other, she started the long climb home. By early afternoon the strength of the sun was already beginning to wane.

Nina had grown tall during the summer. She had begun to menstruate in the spring, and now, although she was taller and slimmer, was beginning to round out in the bosom, buttocks, and thighs. Even though Harriet had let down the hem of her dress and had inserted panels of cloth from other worn-out dresses down the sides in order to accommodate Nina's budding womanliness, still her dress revealed more early bloom than it concealed. In a few days she would be twelve years old. As she toiled up the mountain with her sack and her pail, she must have been unaware, never having seen herself in a mirror, of how appealing a figure she was.

Any mother, when her first little girl shows unmistakable signs of becoming a woman, experiences a faint dismay, a subtle pale desolation. It is probably the one moment when a mother is most motherly; that is, most genuinely unselfish. Her dismay is entirely for the child who has had the door of childhood closed behind her and will go on, unavoidably uninstructed, into the forever and forever world of adult male-and-female complexities.

The early-October afternoon was changing to dusk when Nina rounded the last curve before the lane to the

tent at the top of the mountain. She was startled to see a
man leaning against the trunk of a tree, but then a horse
snorted a greeting and she recognized Injun Jake's white
mare by the side of the road.

"Oh, Jake, you scared me half to death!" she exclaimed.
"For a minute I thought you were a panther! What are you
doing here?"

"My mom's dead," he replied, and a brief tremor con-
torted his face and slightly shook his strong, square body.

"Oh, Jake, I'm so sorry! What happened? When did she
die? Why didn't you come for us to help?"

"Last week," Jake said. "I dint know she was sick. She
said she was tarred and her heart hurt, and she went to bed.
Morning she was dead. I buried her back of the house. Now
I come for you. I take you home with me."

Nina was startled. In her first rush of sympathy she had
moved toward him. At first sight of her, he had pulled
himself away from the tree and walked toward her. They
were standing face to face. There was something in his eyes
that was strange and new, and Nina tensed with alarm.

"I can't go home with you." Her voice was sharp. "I have
to take care of my mother and sister."

Before she could say more, his arms were around her,
pinning her arms and her sack and her pail to her sides. He
pulled her roughly to him until her face was buried in his
shirt against his hairless, stalwart chest. She said to me
years later that he smelled awful. She also said, "I learned
about men from him."

I was shocked.

"Oh, no, Mother! He didn't! He couldn't! Not a twelve-
year-old child! Mother! No!"

And my mother, who by then had spent a lifetime dealing with the joys and sorrows, physical and spiritual, of the
sexual encounter between males and females, blushed like

a twelve-year-old child.

"I didn't mean *that!*" she exclaimed. "Of course Jake wouldn't harm me! I only meant that then was the first time I knew men were made differently, physically, from women."

I was so relieved that I had to laugh. This made my mother grow more red with annoyance. She hadn't meant her story to be funny. And of course it wasn't funny for either Jake or Nina.

Jake's Indian mother had raised her baby to manhood by herself. To have found a hovel and to have successfully provided for her child until he was old enough to help them both was a triumph of love and responsibility. And when she died, the shock for Jake must have been acute. When he wrapped her in a blanket and buried her, coffinless, in a grave he dug himself, he buried the only person in the world to whom he had been of real importance. He must have been dreadfully lonely, and in the dark of that night his mind surely groped here and there for some solution to his need. It was natural he should think of Nina. They had worked in the fields together. He knew she was a deft and willing worker. He had enjoyed her kindness and her laughter and her songs. He must have known, being a normal young male, that she was nubile. It could have come to him as a revelation that near at hand was the answer to the terrible vacuum of his irretrievable loss.

So he had come to claim his bride. While he waited by the wagon road through the long October day, it must have occurred to him that a wife can offer some basic and important pleasures that a mother cannot. Erotic fantasy is not a privilege of the civilized and wellborn alone. As Nina stood before him in her too-tight dress, her face full of the first friendly sympathy for him that he'd seen since his mother was tired and went to bed to die, his loneliness and fear, and his manhood, rose up in him. He clasped to him his self-chosen child bride who was going to make everything all right for him again. And so the child learned from him that men are made differently from women and that this difference is capable of magnificent erection. The child reacted as any young animal reacts to complete surprise: She froze into rigid immobility.

Poor Jake! He had embraced a living girl and found himself holding a steel wire. In a moment he released Nina and stepped back, puzzled by such a reaction to simple passion and simple need. Nina's good right arm, unfettered, swung in a wide arc, and the milk pail at the end of her arm caught Jake on the side of the head. The milk-can top flew off. The butter popped out and rolled into a wagon rut. Milk cascaded over them both. Jake staggered back and sat down. I expect he was dazed by the blow. A two-gallon can full of milk and butter swung by a strong girl free to use the simple principle of centrifugal force is apt to be stunning. Had it been, however, a blow from anyone or anything else, Jake would have been back on his feet instantly, big, strong young savage that he was. But we all know from personal experience that the most disorienting shock comes not from a physical blow but from simple, trusting expectation rejected by someone in whom we have placed candid, and illogical, faith. And so it must have been for him, because he sat by the side of the wagon trail while Nina raced to the tent lane, ran down it, and began to scream for her mother.

Harriet went pale with worry and anger. She must have been appalled when her older daughter began to menstruate. She had, after all, given up all the sensual pleasures of the world for the Lord's sake, not only for herself but for her children. It must have seemed to her a gross injustice that the Lord would allow ordinary sexual maturing to occur, as though Harriet's sacrifice had been somehow unobserved. And for the Lord to have allowed a sinful, lecherous, unsaved, and unwashed half-breed to propose marriage (or its facsimile) to a twelve-year-old child must have made her really angry. The storm broke over Nina's head. I doubt if there are many child psychologists who would recommend this method of dealing with the shocks of puberty, but it certainly had the value of taking Nina's mind completely away from her fright and astonishment.

"I've tried to tell you we must stay away from these ignorant, stubborn mountain people. They will not listen to God's Word. I've tried to tell it to them, but they laugh behind my back. Can't you understand they are not the kind of people you can make your friends? You dare not make friends of the world. If they will not listen to or obey God's law, then they will drag you down to their level and you will be like them. If the world loves you it is because you are one of them. Jesus said, 'Because ye are not of this world, but I have chosen you out of this world, therefore the world hateth you.' So when men want you, beware! It is a sign you are not following Jesus."

This shift of emphasis in a discussion between an adult and a child is the worst kind of motherliness—that is to say, an unfair weapon used against a child who hasn't yet learned that no value can be derived from a discussion that has been artificially shifted from a real and present problem to general intellectual concepts. It is a mother's most effective and damaging device to hide her own inadequacies. Some children never learn how to cope with this maternal trickery, and these children end up pale, frightened, inadequate adults.

Nina gathered her wits together in order to reap some comfort and knowledge from this oblique by-pass.

"Do you mean that if someone likes me and speaks kindly

to me, and they're not Adventists, I'm not either?" she asked. "Why must we be hated to be good?"

"Can't you understand, child? The struggle is not between us and these people. It is between Satan and God. Jesus was persecuted, spat upon, reviled, and cruelly treated. If we follow Him, we will be, too. If we are not, then we can be sure we are not following Him. The servant is not greater than his Lord. They hated Him. They will hate us."

"Why? Why?" demanded Nina, all involved now in this theological discussion. "Old Wally likes me. He laughs at what I say. Mary and Booby like me. Jake likes me," she faltered momentarily, "except there is something wrong with him today. Why do they have to hate me?"

"Now, that's just it," said Harriet, triumphantly. "You should not be saying things to make worldly people laugh. You should be praying unceasingly, and thinking of how to tell them about the Truth!"

"Why do we have to have a God who doesn't want us to be happy or comfortable? I hate Him. I don't want to be saved! I want to live in a house and eat at a table and go to school and be a doctor!" Nina was carried away by nervous tension. "I wish the whole crowd had been drowned in the Red Sea! Then the rest of the Bible would never have been written and we would be home safe with Daddy!"

Harriet became even whiter. She had successfully avoided any discussion of sex, only to find herself listening to heresy.

Serves her right!

Nina crept away to sit by the Sinking Spring, fully expecting to be struck dead by the hand of God.

...13

The next morning Harriet sent Nina over the ridge to the Hurd farm to arrange with John Hurd to bring a horse and wagon and an extra horse to carry their belongings into Waterville as soon as a reply came from Harriet's appeal for house room for the winter. She then made over two of her own dresses for Nina, sewing entirely by hand. One, my mother said, was a very fine gingham, and the other a fine delaine with matching silk braid. They were, Nina thought, the most beautiful dresses in the world.

The hard, ringing October frosts began all at once, and the leaves turned. Nina's feet became frostbitten, and chilblains made her feet and ankles burn and itch. Harriet boiled up potato peelings, and when the brew was cool enough Nina plunged in her feet and ankles, happily squeezing the soft, warm, slippery skins between her toes. When the brew became tepid, she plunged her feet into a bucket of ice-cold spring water while Harriet reheated the potatoes. After four or five shifts between hot pail and cold pail, the itching stopped. Nina lingered in the hot-potato pail, feeling like a coddled princess, tenderly ministered to.

A week later, Nina went to Waterville for the mail and to arrange with Dave Lovett to store the tent gear for the winter. There were two letters, one from Philadelphia and one from Williamsport. Nina raced home in a glow of expectation. Harriet read the letters aloud. The letter from Williamsport, from the church, was loving. With great tact and respect for human dignity Brother Leeland urged her to come to them. The children, he said, could help in the household before and after school; Harriet would be a blessing in the Work.

The letter from Philadelphia was specific. The aunt, who with her half of Harriet's father's money had been able, through her husband, to make more money, was old and widowed. She felt it to be her duty to help Harriet, but she could not imagine living a normal, retiring life with two children underfoot. She would be willing to take in Harriet and one child, but no more than one. She had enclosed two tickets to Philadelphia, one full fare and one half fare.

Harriet prayed briefly for guidance and then announced that she and Dorothy would go to Philadelphia and Nina would go to Williamsport.

I wonder what it would be like to be rejected totally by one's mother when one is twelve years old. Most of us at that age have had moments of fear that Mother might love someone else more than oneself. But we bury the fear, because to be sure that such a thing could be is worse than to live with the fear itself. For Nina, it must have been the end of hope. Did the tears that gushed like a spring freshet from her eyes more than sixty years later come really from sorrow that her mother's baby died, leaving her mother comfortless, or did they come from a pool of despair formed that day when she learned that she herself, no matter how hard she tried, was never to be her mother's baby, ever? It was perhaps a measure of Nina's defeat that she didn't weep, didn't argue, didn't say anything, but began, the next morning, to gather her meager clothes together to pack in a cardboard box tied shut by a string.

Only two trains passed through Waterville each day: the milk train at eight in the morning and the train at five o'clock in the afternoon. Both of these went to Williamsport on their way to other places. It would be impossible, in view of the heavy morning frost and the late rising of the October sun, to make the three-hour walk in time to catch the milk train. Nina kissed her mother and her sister and was ready to leave soon after their noon lunch. She had enough money left over from the chestnuts to buy her ticket on the train. The address of Brother Leeland in Williamsport was tucked in her pocket.

"I wish you had shoes and stockings," Harriet said. "It's so cold!"

"Oh, I'll run fast. I can stop often to warm my feet under my dress. Don't worry. I don't need shoes. The sun is out and it's never so windy over the cutoff as it is here. Mr. Hurd will come for you tomorrow. There's enough food 'til then."

Nina took one last look at her mother and sister and left the tent. She ran down the lane and was part way down the mountain before she huddled in a sheltered place to wrap the skirt of her new dress around her ice-cold feet. She arrived in Waterville more than an hour before the train was due. The station, which was opened only just before a train came in, was locked tight, so she went across to the general store to say goodbye to Dave Lovett. He was taking a day off for hunting, however, and Mr. Fry, the same Mr. Fry who owned the shack in Rattlesnake Run where the counterfeiters were squatting, was minding the store.

"Well, well!" he said. "Looks as if you was going somewhere."

"Yes, I'm going away to school in Williamsport. I have the address written down here in my pocket." She patted her pocket to hear the paper rattle. "I can ask where it is when I get off the train. It's only a block from the station, and Mother says it's a big building. It's a publishing house where they print religious tracts and the *Keystone Gleaner*— that's a paper that's sent to all the church people. The Leelands live next door. I'm to live with them and go to school."

"Well, well!" said Mr. Fry, somewhat overwhelmed by all this unexpected information. "That's nice. You ought to go to school, and tain't safe for any of you up in the woods. Where's your pa? Why don't he come and get you?" At the sight of sudden tears in her eyes he went on hurriedly, "Thar now, don't cry. I didn't go to hurt your feelings. He'll come for you when he can. Whar's your shoes?"

Nina was abashed. "I don't have any."

"Well, come on back to where the shoes is, and we'll see if we can't find some to fit." Mr. Fry was already walking toward the back of the store.

"I don't need shoes," Nina said quickly. "And besides, we don't take charity."

Mr. Fry turned. "Charity! Who said charity? Dave wouldn't pay me long to mind his store if I give his things away. I'll fit you with shoes and stockings and I'll give you a paper writ legal that tells what you owe, and when you're done with school and workin', you can send Dave the money. He'll need it more then, anyways."

Nina was entranced with such a transaction. "That would be splendid! Do you have low shoes, pretty black ones?"

"No." Mr. Fry hardened his heart. "You need high shoes for winter, and rubbers too. It's going to be a snowy winter, and you'll want warm feet. . . . Goddamn it! Your feet are all frostbitten. What in hell does your mother mean, letting you go like that?"

Nina looked up, startled. "Oh, Mr. Fry! Don't swear. That's wicked. My mother's all right, and so are my feet. It just got cold all of a sudden."

"Of course it did. I didn't mean to swear; it just popped out. Now let's try on a pair for size."

Warmly shod in black cotton stockings and stout high-buttoned shoes and rubbers, with a cunning little shoebuttoner in her pocket, she climbed aboard the train. As it rattled down the mountain through the early dusk, lamps were being lit in the scattered farmhouses along the way. Never had the child felt so alone as in that loneliest hour of the day when families gather together against the coming of night. Panic rose inside her. This is as bad as walking past a panther, she said to herself. She forced herself to sit quietly; she was afraid that if she moved at all, she would fight to get off the train to go back to the tent and to her mother.

The train conductor who had sold her her ticket came back and sat beside her and talked to her. He was a Williamsport man, and even knew the building where she was going.

"You just stand still when you get off the train," he said. "As soon as the other passengers are off, I'll take you to the publishing house. We'll find the Leelands together." Panic subsided in her breast.

"Thank you," she said gratefully. "Mother has told me always to ask a man who wears a uniform if I need help. She said a uniformed man always directs girls safely." She smiled at him brilliantly.

Comforted now, she rode through the darkness into a new life.

PART TWO

"*Work, for the night is coming.*"

...1

Accompanied by the train conductor, Nina found the church printing plant with no difficulty. Next to the plant was a large, wood-frame house, gabled, and fronted by such a narrow, high-roofed porch that the spaced supports, slender and plain, looked ludicrously delicate against the bulk of the house itself. It was a house whose destiny was inherent in its size; it would later become a boardinghouse. Later still, it would be bought for the value of the land by a real-estate developer who would demolish the house and with it even the memory of the lives that had been lived inside. There was lamplight glowing from the windows.

"Well, Nina," said the conductor, "I guess you're safe now. I'll have to get back to the train. I hope you enjoy school as much as you think you will. I never liked it much myself, but maybe I should have thought about school differently. Too late now. Goodbye and good luck!" They shook hands warmly and Nina watched him as he walked through the front gate and merged into the night. She climbed the steps, crossed the porch, and knocked at the door.

Nina was to remember for years how frightened she was as she stood there in the dark, waiting for the door to open. When Sister Leeland stood in the opened doorway, a lamp held high, Nina's spirits lifted as she realized that she had seen this woman before at the long-ago Camp Meeting. Sister Leeland was a link, tenuous enough and frail, with some known part of her past life. All was not lost.

"I'm Nina Mae Case," the child said. "You offered to take us all in but my mother and sister are going to Philadelphia and I've come to live with you."

"Gracious sakes!" Mrs. Leeland exclaimed. "Why didn't your mother let me know? How brave of you to come all that way alone! You're welcome, Nina Mae, and there's plenty of room. Myra! Fred!" she called, drawing Nina into the front hall. "Come fast. Here's Nina Mae come to live with us!" Such a welcome strengthens the frightened heart.

Myra came quietly into the hall. She was Nina's age, but she was big and plump, with fat blond braids tied with big, bright ribbons. She had a habit of turning her head away to the side so that she looked at others with a sidelong glance that made her seem sly.

Fred bounced into the entrance hall with the flopsy-mopsy gait of an overgrown puppy. He was seven years old, and to him everything in life was fun and excitement.

"Myra," said Sister Leeland, "take Nina Mae up to the attic bedroom and then show her where to wash up. Nina Mae, when you're ready, come down and we'll fix you some supper. My goodness! It's past eight o'clock. You must be starved."

Myra led the way as Nina followed wearily. They went up a long flight of stairs, turned down a long hall, and at the end went through a door to a closed stairway leading to the attic. At the top of the stairway was a vast attic with a small room partitioned off from the rest of the space. Nina looked around her room. How beautiful! she thought. There was a cot with a flowered counterpane that exactly matched the flowered washstand pitcher and slop jar; there was a chair with a cushion on the seat; there was a small table with a lace cover and a Bible on it; there was a motto on the wall, "The Kingdom of God is come nigh unto you," and on the dormer windows there were crisp white curtains. Directly opposite the door was a dresser with a mirror. This was the first time in three years that Nina had

seen her own face except for the times she caught a dim
reflection in Sinking Spring. She was entranced. The fat
blonde girl standing next to her was giving her a blue,
sidelong glance. What a beautiful room!

"This is your bedroom," Myra said, "and the bathroom
is at the end of the hall downstairs, at the back. Come down
when you're ready." She set the oil lamp on the table next
to the Bible. She slid out of the door and flew down the dark
enclosed staircase as though she were pursued by demons.

Nina sat down on the chair. Suddenly she realized that
her feet were burning beyond endurance. She pulled off
her rubbers and unbuttoned her sturdy shoes. She pulled
off her long black stockings. She was very tired. The emotional strain of parting, the seven-mile walk, the train trip,
and the strangeness of being in a room with a real bed at
just the hour her mother and sister must be settling down
in their fragrant hemlock boughs, all combined to drain her
of strength. She crept to the cot thinking, I'll just lie down
for a moment to rest, and when she woke she was undressed and under the covers, the sun was shining in the
window, and from far away she heard voices and pots clink-
ing.

She jumped out of bed and almost fell down as she
tripped over the voluminous folds of a strange nightgown,
obviously made for a large woman. The ruffles at the wrists
covered her hands and the ruffle at the hem trailed behind
her like a wedding train. She was so appalled at having
slept so long that she had little time to be amazed at her
nightdress. She crept down the stairs to the washroom, fled
back to her room, dressed as carefully and as quickly as she
could, combed and braided her long dark hair, and in bare
feet made her way to the ground floor. The rattling of pots
and pans led her through the dining room, where the table
was set, the place settings covered over with a large white

cloth. She went down two steps into the kitchen. Sister Leeland looked up from the stove where she was stirring cooked cereal in a large double boiler. She smiled kindly.

"Did you get your sleep out, Nina Mae?" she asked. "You really were tired. We tried to wake you to give you something to eat, but you wouldn't wake up, so I put you to bed. I couldn't find a nightgown in your box, so I used one of mine."

"My nightgowns are all worn out, so I sleep in my skin."

"Good gracious! How awful! Don't mention such a thing to Myra or Fred."

"It's not so awful. In fact, in some ways it's better than sleeping in a gown." Nina was always candid. "I can curl up with myself with nothing pulling on me. Sometimes when it's cold, though, I wish I had fur like a squirrel."

Sister Leeland was not mollified. "How awful! Don't tell anybody! In this house we all wear nightclothes. You can use mine until we can make some for you. But goodness, child! Where are your shoes and stockings?"

"Oh!" Nina was amazed. "Should I wear them here in the house? I was saving them for school."

Just then they both heard the rest of the household coming downstairs and a deep male voice calling to Myra and Fred to come immediately for morning worship. Mrs. Leeland took off her apron and hung it on a hook by the kitchen door. She smoothed her hair. "We'll talk after breakfast. Come along to the parlor for worship. You'll meet the rest of the family."

Brother Leeland sat in a straight-backed armchair, looking, Nina thought, like King David. He was a tall, lean man with black hair, blue eyes, and a stern black beard. Millie, the spinster secretary of the Williamsport Church Conference, sat in a low rocking chair near the organ. Millie was tall, pale, and slender, with a bad complexion. Next to her sat Mr. Gibson, the printer, and next to him, Sister Munson, the Bible worker. Then Myra and Fred. Sister Leeland introduced Nina to the others and they took their places, Nina next to Fred. Mrs. Leeland completed the circle.

"Millie," asked Brother Leeland solemnly, "will you play for us?"

Millie went to the organ and they all sang a hymn.

"We will now read the eighth chapter of Deuteronomy," announced Brother Leeland. Fred was fidgeting in his chair. "Fred," said his father sternly, "sit still. Read the first two verses." Fred read haltingly. As he read, Mrs. Leeland said in an anxious aside to Nina, "Tomorrow bring your Bible down with you."

"That's all right," Nina whispered, "I know this all by heart."

When Fred finished his two verses, Nina took up the theme with the next two verses, speaking softly in her clear young voice.

"And he humbled thee, and suffered thee to hunger, and fed thee with manna, which thou knewest not, nor did thy fathers know; that he might make thee know that man doth not live by bread only, but by every word that proceedeth out of the mouth of the Lord doth man live. Thy raiment waxed not old upon thee, neither did thy foot swell, these forty years."

When Harriet and the children had studied these verses on the mountain, Nina had pointed out to her mother that the children of Israel, in their wilderness, were lucky indeed; Nina's raiment had worn out in less than three years and her feet were often swollen. Harriet found the comparison presumptuous.

Brother Leeland, unwaveringly solemn, commended Nina for needing no written text for her verses. He then said, "Let us pray," and they all knelt on the floor in front of their chairs. He prayed in a loud bishop's voice for each one of those kneeling before him, calling each by name. Then they all rose and Millie played one verse of "Work, for the night is coming when man works no more."

Mrs. Leeland motioned to Myra and Nina to follow her.

"You girls remove the cloth from the table, and then come and help me in the kitchen."

The children, one at each end of the table, lifted and folded the spotless white cloth that covered the breakfast place settings. They poured fresh water into the adults' glasses and milk in the children's mugs. They carried in a bowl of fruit and a bowl of hot cereal for each plate. Nina thought how fine it was to have so much for breakfast. She carried in two platters of thick brown slices of toast, and all was ready. The household gathered for breakfast.

There was little conversation. Millie spoke only when the printer or Brother Leeland asked her a question. Brother Leeland and Mr. Gibson talked of the work they would do that day at the office. Sister Munson spoke not at all. Mrs. Leeland busied herself with extra servings and with keeping Fred sitting in his chair. Nina, uncertain of what to do, watched the others and did what they did. She helped herself to toast when one of the big platters was passed to her side of the table, but turned it timidly around in her hand until she could see how the others ate it. Each one broke off a piece and began to chew. Nina laughed. Everyone stopped chewing at once.

"Well!" said Brother Leeland sternly. "What happened to you?"

"Nothing, really," Nina answered meekly, in an agony of embarrassment.

"Nothing? Nonsense! People don't laugh at nothing."

"It was only that you all made such a funny noise chewing this hard toast that you sounded like Old Wally's horses

in the barn chewing their corn. It made me laugh, remembering Old Wally's horses. They were always so serious
about eating."

No one smiled. Millie looked at her plate. Mr. Gibson
looked out of the window.

"That is not funny," announced Brother Leeland, "and
little girls should be seen and not heard."

Breakfast continued. From then on, Nina ate her meals
without speaking unless she was spoken to and without
laughing at the table, which the family never did.

That first morning in the kitchen after breakfast Sister
Leeland said, "Since today is Friday, Nina Mae, I think
you'd better not start to school. Wait until Monday. Today
you can get acquainted with your duties here, and get used
to the house so you won't feel strange." Nina, who had
already waited for twelve years to go to school, was willing
to wait until Monday. After they had washed the breakfast
dishes and cleaned the kitchen until it gleamed in the
morning light, and after Myra and Fred had left for school,
Mrs. Leeland and Nina went to the attic bedroom to look
over Nina's clothes.

"From what I saw last night," Mrs. Leeland said, "you
don't have many clothes. We will have to think what to do.
By the way, dear, what shall we call you? Are you Nina
Mae or just Nina?"

"Oh, please call me just plain Nina," she said. "That's all
I've ever been called and it would seem more like home to
me."

"Very well, just plain Nina." Sister Leeland laughed.
"Let's look at your clothes."

There weren't many. Nina had on the same dress she had
worn on the train—a black gingham made-over dress. She
had the beautiful blue delaine for the Sabbath, a white
embroidered blouse and blue skirt for school. She had a

pitiful handful of underthings, one pair of black stockings, her shoes, and her rubbers.

"That's not much," observed Mrs. Leeland, "but it will have to do for now. Maybe the sewing circle of the church can make over some dresses for you."

"Oh, no!" Nina was shocked. "There are many people in the world with less than this. The sewing circle mustn't waste its time on me. I can wash my clothes at night." She was so distressed that Sister Leeland patted her hand and agreed that, with the addition of some nightgowns, there really were enough clothes.

"But," Sister Leeland said, "you must wear shoes all of the time, except in your own room."

The pattern of daily living in the household was well organized, and between Friday and Monday mornings Nina became part of a routine that was not to vary for the entire time she lived with the Leelands. It is to the credit of these kindly people that no one under their roof, spinster, widow, or orphan, was exploited. Nina was to work hard, but Myra shared all her tasks equally. The women and girls rose at five-thirty in the morning and collected the oil lamps, which, when they were blown out at night, were put outside the bedroom doors. Each person had his own particular lamp with its own individual place on the kitchen shelf. Nina, Myra, and Millie washed and refilled the bowls, trimmed the wicks, and washed and polished the chimneys before putting the lamps in order on the shelf. All of the beds were stripped to air. Then came morning worship, and then breakfast. After breakfast the women cleared the table, washed the dishes, and reset the table for dinner, covering the place settings with the big white cloth. They made the beds. The children left for school.

Dinner was at noon. There was only time for Myra and Nina to help serve the meal, eat, and get back to school.

After school they did whatever Mrs. Leeland found for them to do—cleaned cupboards, ironed, beat rugs, dusted. Supper was a light meal, and after evening worship the children did their lessons and went to bed.

An orderly, useful life.

...2

Monday morning came, and Nina was going to school. She woke in a glow of anticipation. After she had washed and dressed, she picked up her own lamp and, on the floor below, the lamp of Brother Gibson, and made her way down to the kitchen. As she reached the dining room she heard Myra sobbing in the kitchen.

"Oh, Mother! I won't take Nina to school. All the girls will laugh at me! She doesn't even know what grade she's in. Maybe they'll put her in the first grade and everyone will laugh. And she looks so funny—no hat, no ribbons in her hair. I won't do it, and you can't make me!"

"Now, dear, don't be silly," said Sister Leeland soothingly. "Of course you must take her to school. She can wear some of your ribbons."

"I won't let her. Everyone will know they're mine."

"Land's sake, Myra. Enough of this nonsense. You must conquer your pride."

As Myra drew in her breath to bully her mother, Nina marched into the kitchen with her lamps. She put them down with a thud on the wooden kitchen table. She turned to Myra, scorn in her eyes.

"I can find my way. You needn't take me to school. I can take care of myself. I don't need you. I won't walk to school with you today, or ever." And she never did, although after a few days they always walked home from school together. Pride can be modified in many directions without being humbled.

Nina took a lamp chimney and turned abruptly to the basin of warm, soapy water in the sink. All of her glow was drained away. The long-wished-for day, the first day of school, was in ruins because of hair ribbons. She didn't worry about what grade she would be put in; she knew it wouldn't be the first grade, and any reasonable grade would be school. But her heart was sore and swollen in her chest to know she would look funny without a hat and without hair ribbons. She wanted so much to look ordinary, to take her place unobtrusively in the magic world of public school.

When the after-breakfast chores were finished, she slipped out of the house and followed other children down the street and around corners until she reached the main street of the town. There the children seemed to scatter. She didn't know whom to follow. There was a big policeman directing traffic in the center of the main street, so she went out to him.

"Please, could you tell me the way to school?" she asked.

There wasn't much traffic, as we know traffic today, but there were horse-drawn drays, carriages for the well-to-do, bicycles, surreys, and horsemen on their morning trips. The policeman changed his stop-and-go arrows and turned to Nina.

"What school do you want?" he asked. "The grammar school is over that way and the high school is down that street four blocks."

"The high school, I guess." Nina was doubtful. All she knew was that one day, after she was ten years old, her mother had said, "You're in high school now, Nina." When the policeman changed his arrows again, she went down the street four blocks and there was the school.

She stood forlorn and alone in the big entrance hall. All of the other children were rushing about, greeting each other, pushing and laughing and moving with confidence and purpose. All of the girls wore hair ribbons.

A teacher, passing by, noticed Nina standing quietly against the wall. "Are you a new student?" he asked.

"Yes, sir, and I don't know where I belong, or what to do."

"Come with me," he said. He took Nina to the office of the principal. There was no one in the office, but the teacher told Nina to sit down, and Mr. Worley, the principal, would be there soon. Nina sat.

In a few minutes Mr. Worley came in. He smiled at Nina in exactly the way a school principal who likes young people should smile. He asked her where she had been to school.

"I've never been to school. My mother taught me at home."

Just then a teacher came in. Mr. Worley and the teacher conferred together about everyday morning problems. Then Mr. Worley asked Nina to sit down and wait while he rang the bells and got the classes under way. As he went out of the door he turned.

"Why don't you, in the meantime, go over to those shelves of books, pick out the books you've studied, and put them on the table. Then we'll have some idea of where we are." He smiled again, and Nina was sure his plan would work. She went to the shelves and was at once absorbed in the books. How wonderful! All those books! There were many she had never seen before, but there were many, many old friends. She peeked into some and patted others as she put them on the table. English, American history, ancient history, world history, geography, Latin, algebra, advanced algebra, trigonometry, geometry, physiology, French, English novels, American essays—so many friends! The shelves were sparse and the table was piled high with books when Mr. Worley finally returned.

"Well, well! Quite an array," he said, looking at her curiously. "Sit here by my desk and tell me about yourself. How old are you?"

"I'm twelve years old." Nina felt very much at home with this man. He looked at her with interest, the way one person should look at another person. He reached over to the table and picked up a book at random. It was a volume of poems by Catullus, in Latin. He flipped it open and asked her to translate a poem on that page.

Nina was pleased. She had never seen a whole volume of poems by Catullus, but he had been included in a fat volume of Roman poets she had studied, and this particular poem was one she liked, because it was so gay.

> *Give me a thousand kisses, and then another thousand!*
> *Let us count the advice of our elders*
> *Just to the worth of a cent.*
> *Give me a thousand kisses!* . . .

Mr. Worley smiled back at Nina as she finished.

"You like to read, don't you?" he asked.

"Oh, yes. Especially stories in English. I read all my mother's books many times, but one summer day I found an abandoned house. The whole house had been papered inside with newspapers—the *Pennsylvania Grit.* They all had wonderful continued stories. I almost had to stand on my head to read some of the pages. The worst of it was that after searching all the walls and ceilings I sometimes couldn't find the end of the stories, and sometimes I couldn't even find the beginning. Yes, I like to read. You have many books here I haven't read yet."

"Are you sure you've read all those books on the table?" Mr. Worley asked doubtfully. As Nina nodded, he picked up a pointer from the desk. "Suppose you point out Afghanistan on that map and tell me what you know about the country."

"I'd love to. I lived there for almost a week."

"What?" Mr. Worley was astonished. More than astonished; distrustful. His face began to harden with distrust.

"Oh, I'm sorry." Nina blushed. "Not really. I didn't really live in Afghanistan. Whenever we studied a country, Mother had us live there. We dressed and lived, during geography lesson, as we read how they dressed and lived there, and she asked us all about the country. We did that with all the different countries, and we couldn't come back to America until we knew all about the major cities, the capital, the population, agriculture, industries, and folklore. We lived longest in Egypt, because we had to live in different periods. We were the children of all the separate dynasties."

"That *is* interesting," said Mr. Worley, his face all kindness. "Your mother must be a remarkable woman. Now it's almost dinnertime. Come back here to the office after dinner and we'll try to finish the examination and place you where you belong."

Nina hurried home. She was busy in the kitchen helping dish up the dinner when Myra came in.

"Where did they put you?" Myra asked.

"Nowhere, yet. I am to go back after dinner to finish being examined."

"Haven't they sent you over to the grade school?"

"Not yet." Nina spoke pleasantly. In her heart there was a quiet, unruffled place that was Mr. Worley.

In the principal's office after dinner, Mr. Worley had two

teachers with him. They asked many questions. They gave Nina problems in geometry and algebra and trigonometry to solve. They had her translate French exercises. They asked her about events and dates in history. They were all friendly, good-humored, and fascinated. Nina enjoyed the afternoon. She didn't feel on trial; they were all working together to find a place for her.

Shortly before three o'clock the principal said, "Come with me," and all four of them, Mr. Worley, Nina, and the two teachers, went into the assembly room. All of the high school was already seated there. A hush settled over the room as they filed down the aisle to the front of the hall. For the first time since the opening of school Nina thought about how she looked. They went to the front row, where Nina and the two teachers sat down. Mr. Worley stood before the asssembled students and teachers. He explored general school problems and projects with the student body. Then he said:

"I want to introduce to you now a little girl whom I am proud to know. She is twelve years old, and she is being admitted into the senior class of this high school. She has already done most of the work of the senior class, but there are some gaps in her education we can fill this year, and she needs to be a regular member of a public school in order to have a diploma. She has never been to school before because she has been tutored at home, so she feels strange. I hope the girls in her class, and the girls her own age, will really try to welcome her and help her feel one of us. You can trust me when I say that she is worth being friends with. Nina, will you stand up?"

Nina stood up, but she was unable to turn around to face the school. All that the students saw, as they clapped, was her narrow dark head and her long braids held in neat order by thread wound around the tips. Everyone clapped boisterously, partly for the phenomenon that was Nina and partly because the school day was over.

At the close of the general assembly, girls, led by Genevieve Timbell, the senior beauty and leader of the in-group, gathered around Nina. The girls vied with each other to ask her questions and exclaim over her. They walked together slowly out of the school in a group, and down to the main street of town. There they scattered, chirping and shrilling goodbyes and see-you-tomorrows and let's-all-get-together-Sunday-afternoon-for-some-fun. Nina walked sedately around the corner and, when she was out of sight of the rest, ran the rest of the way home in a burst of happiness and excitement. She fairly danced across the narrow porch and down the hall to the kitchen. In the kitchen, Myra was crying.

"Why didn't you tell me you were so smart?" Myra burst out when Nina appeared.

Nina stood in the doorway at the top of the steps into the kitchen. Her excitement died, and she considered Myra thoughtfully.

The episode of Nina's first day at school was to become one of our favorite stories. When we were children, it never failed to shock us deeply that Myra hadn't wanted to take Mother to school. We felt a personal triumph when Nina was put in the senior class of high school. But it was the final scene, Myra undone by the sin of pride, that delighted us most. We could believe without question that right always wins, goodness and industry are always rewarded, and the mean of spirit always end up crying in the kitchen.

"I'm sorry, Myra," Nina said, "that I make you worry so much. This morning you cried because you thought I was stupid, and now you're crying because you think I'm smart. I'm not smart; my mother made me work very hard. I thought you'd be glad I wasn't put in the first grade."

Myra sniffled. Sister Leeland said that they were all glad for Nina. She alternately patted first one child and then the other, unable to decide which one needed mothering most. Brother Leeland, at evening worship, commented kindly on the success of Nina's examinations. He looked sternly at Myra as he said, " 'Man looketh on the outward appearance, but the Lord looketh on the heart.' "

...3

Nina read everything she could find to read. Late at night her lamp burned, with no one in her attic to say she must blow it out to sleep. One Sunday morning, having finished reading all the books she had brought home from school on Friday, she wandered over to the printing plant next door to see what there was there to read. In the big sorting room she found a large stack of little books. They were children's books called *The House We Live In*. It occurred to her that they were an ideal size to put in children's Christmas stockings. She had been trying to think of a way to earn money for underwear and a warm coat for winter. She took a copy of the little book to Brother Leeland, who was in the printing plant office. If the books were not already ordered by some group, she asked, could she try to sell them in the neighborhood to earn some money? Brother Leeland thought about the proposal soberly. Yes, he decided, she could try. But for each one she sold, she must give a small part of the money to the plant for printing costs. He warned her that Williamsport was not a town noted for its reading public. The one bookstore in town had a hard time keeping its doors open. It would be even more difficult to sell a sectarian religious book door to door. But she could try.

Nina proposed that she be excused from her regular household chores for two hours after school every day. Brother Leeland consulted with his wife at dinner that noon, and it was agreed that Nina would be released from duty from then until Christmas, or for as long as she worked on the new project. On Monday afternoon she gathered up an armload of the little books and started out. In two hours she had sold all of the books.

Every day after school, regardless of the weather, she spent two hours peddling the little books, and every day she sold all she could carry. By Christmastime she had enough money for a coat, for material for a new skirt and blouse, and for extra underwear. And she had enough left over to send to the general store in Waterville the payment for her shoes, stockings, and rubbers. I expect that Dave Lovett, in Waterville, was surprised to get the money, carefully folded in a paper "writ legal" and signed in Nina's best handwriting, "Paid in full, Nina Mae Case." He was bound to think of her with pleasure, although they were never to meet again.

...4

The class Nina enjoyed the most at school was English composition. She had never had an opportunity to write stories and essays before. Harriet had seen little value in writing. She felt no need to write out her own fantasies; she was much too busy acting them out in real life. But her respect for the printed word was absolute, believing as she did that thoughts great enough to be set in type and bound into books deserved not only preservation but intelligent attention, whether one agreed with those thoughts or not. For Nina, to be encouraged to write down her own stories was both heaven and hell. She had no lack of material; her active, well-stocked mind was crammed with stories, but her idea of punctuation was derived directly from the King James version of the Bible. Such punctuation does not fit in with the average high school teacher's view of humdrum clarity.

She was still too close to her immediate past life in the mountains to write about the actual events that had happened to her. Experiences of the past must be rewritten in the secret mind before they can be told to strangers. Nina's stories were about witches and ghosts, Greek islands and Roman military camps in fearful virgin forests.

Myra and Fred had begun to spend most of their evenings after supper in Nina's attic room, doing their own homework and listening in delicious terror to Nina's latest composition. Nina's fame as a storyteller spread from Myra and Fred, and from her own classwork, until every Sunday afternoon a bevy of girls collected in the attic to listen in on the latest flight of fancy. One Sunday afternoon, someone suggested that they turn the stories into plays and act them out. Week after week, more and more lavish productions were staged, using the stored Seventh-Day Adventist Camp Meeting equipment for props. The attic and the big wooden house echoed with shrieks of laughter and groans of derision.

Sunday, for Brother Leeland, was a working day at the printing plant. One Sunday afternoon, however, he came back to the house early and, hearing unusual noises from the attic, went quietly up the stairs and stood watching the production. When the children finally became aware of an alien presence at the door, he stepped gravely into the attic. There was an apprehensive silence.

"What is the meaning of this? Who suggested doing this worldly thing, having a theater in our own home, playing lies, impossible things, witches and talking trees?"

Myra, who knew that her father must always be answered when he questioned, was the one who spoke. "Nina's doing it, Papa. I was only listening," she said.

Brother Leeland gave his daughter a stern, reproving glance. Even a just man disapproves of stool pigeons. "You children must all go home. Do not come here again. Nina, bring all the wicked plays you have written into the parlor. We will read them over and let the family decide what we must do about it."

He trod heavily down the stairs, followed by the children. Nina was left alone to collect her stories and to meet the household in the parlor.

Brother and Sister Leeland, Millie, Sister Munson, and Brother Gibson were all assembled. Nina took a place in the circle, and Brother Leeland asked her to read her stories aloud. Past the lump in her throat and the tears in her eyes, Nina read. Once, looking up, she caught the trace of a smile on Brother Gibson's face, but it vanished as he gazed carefully out the window.

The decision of the household was that Nina must confess her sin to the Lord so that she might not become the "mother of liars," and she must burn her manuscripts. The tears dried in her eyes and the lump in her breast was replaced by an iron bar of indignation.

"You can't ask me to burn my stories! These are my stories, and you cannot have them to burn. I'm sorry about the plays. I should have asked. I didn't know plays were worldly. But these stories are my own, and you have no right to destroy them."

Brother Leeland was not one to argue principles with a twelve-year-old girl. "You will burn them now," he said. "Go and put them into the stove."

Nina went. With dark rebellion in her heart, she

watched the pages burn and the edges catch fire and a word leap out at her and a word fade into ashes.

This was a Pyrrhic victory for Brother Leeland. I think no one ever in the history of the world has won a lasting victory against ideas unacceptable to him by burning the paper on which the ideas are written. Nina was, after all, her mother's daughter, and she had adopted as her own Harriet's attitude, all the more easily accepted because it had been stated by example rather than discussion, that the written word is sacred and should not be burned up. Phoenixes rise from ashes.

...5

In early May, 1897, after Nina had lived with the Leelands through the long cold winter, the weather turned unseasonably warm. The exuberant rambling roses that rioted over the fences between the front lawns and the tamped-earth sidewalks of Williamsport were all in bloom and the citizens walked slowly in a languid, rose-scented premature summer. At school, the children lazily turned the handles of the pencil sharpeners on the windowsills, dreamily gazing outside at nothing and hearing nothing being said within. No one hurried. No one did anything unexpected. But an event was about to take place that might seem unusual to anyone who has never lived within a close-knit, communal religious cult.

Graduation day was scheduled for mid-June. Nina, who was finishing in one school year the academic requirements that in those days usually took twelve years of formal education to achieve, was about to graduate from high school. Brother Leeland had already written to Harriet for suggestions as to what next might be done with her child. Harriet had not answered his letter. The responsibility of deciding Nina's immediate future had fallen upon Brother Leeland, her guardian by default. He did not take responsibility lightly. At a moment when the coming necessity to make some decision must have been nagging at his mind, he had an offer from a member of the church congregation which would solve the problem of what would become of Nina after graduation. He was not slow to take a manna-from-Heaven view of the proposal, which came from Sister Lightner.

Sister Alice Lightner taught the Seventh-Day Adventist Sabbath School. Myra, Fred, Nina, and the other church children of Williamsport spent every Saturday morning every week of the year with Sister Lightner. She had formed a special relationship with Nina. I know this because Mother once told us that Myra had complained to her parents that Sister Lightner "likes Nina best. She only really talks to Nina, and that's not fair!" Sister Lightner's proposal was that Nina should live with her for the next few years.

Alice Lightner's husband had been a well-to-do convert to the church. Their only child, Will, was five years old when Brother Lightner died in the rose-scented spring of the year. Alice's husband had left enough money to keep his family in modest comfort. Alice planned to return to her home town of Battle Creek, Michigan; she offered to take Nina with her. Nina could help with little Will. Nina's company would be welcome in the long sad evenings ahead. Sister Lightner, moreover, would pay the fees so that Nina could become a day student at Battle Creek College, one of the three Seventh-Day Adventist colleges in the United States in 1897.

Little wonder that Brother Leeland looked favorably on

her proposal. It appeared to be an admirable plan for the child, whose mother had no plan for her at all. If it seems unusual that adults should be handing around among them a child with whom none of them had any legal relationship, it is not uncommon even today for members of a closed religious group to regard each other as an extended family and to put consideration for the good of the cause far above concern for individual preferences, especially those of children. Brother Leeland wrote again to Harriet, this time outlining Sister Lightner's specific proposal.

The day before graduation, a letter from Harriet arrived. She approved of the plan. She herself was not going back to the mountain. She had already sent for her possessions stored in Dave Lovett's store. She could not take Nina. She was, as they knew, a penniless dependent. May God reward them for their kindness and may they all be happy in the Lord.

Only after Harriet's letter had arrived was Nina consulted about her wishes. She was ecstatic. No grief for her lost mother diluted her joy. She would go on to school and somehow she would become a doctor. Harriet was unimportant. The rejector was rejected. Freud once said, "When I have forgiven a man everything, I am through with him." I know nothing more of Harriet except that she left the Seventh-Day Adventist Church and that she died old. "For what is your life? It is even a vapour, that appeareth for a little time, and then vanisheth away."

...6

In Battle Creek, Michigan, in early July, Nina dressed for her first day of college. Sister Lightner had made her a new dress—dark blue with rows of red rickrack at the high neck, at the neat, close-fitting vee of the bodice, at the cuffs, and around the folds of the hem, which just cleared the floor. The dark bright blue made brilliant her pale clear-blue eyes. She walked the few blocks between their apartment and the Seventh-Day Adventist Battle Creek Sanitarium, and there was the college. It was only one big old building on the sweeping lawns of the sanitarium, but for Nina the lawns were a campus solely designed to make her college as significant and imposing as a college should be. I doubt if anyone, ever, found the day of matriculation in college so completely satisfying. "Doth not wisdom cry? . . . She crieth at the gates, at the entry . . . at the coming in at the doors." Nina, still twelve years old, entered the doors.

The summer session and the first full year of Battle Creek College that began in late September continued to be satisfactory. In English composition Nina could now, from a point of some perspective, write about life in the Pennsylvania forest. She wrote about the fire-killed ghost forest on Brown's Run. She wrote about an old soldier's funeral, and this essay was read by her English teacher one morning at chapel services. Nina was enthralled when at times his voice broke and the listening students sat in total silence. Words are powerful, she thought. And words are free; anyone can use them.

I don't know what old soldier's funeral she attended up there in the mountains. There are so many things about those years I'll never know. What I do know about Nina's life comes in part from the voluminous notes Nina herself kept. She was an inveterate writer. All her life she wrote things down and she never threw a note away. Many years later she handed me boxes and boxes of notes: shoeboxes; old-fashioned shirt boxes that once contained a dozen collarless shirts and a dozen stiff collars in their own separate compartments; cardboard cartons stamped with brand names of wares no longer found on the market. One box contained reminiscences that had been typed by a grateful patient, which must have been Nina's attempt late in a busy life to bring order out of chaos.

The most important source of what I know comes, of course, from my own memories of what she said to me and to my sisters. When, later, Nina was to become the sole support of her own three little girls, she earned our daily bread as a doctor in an era when professional women were still unacceptable to those with enough money to pay fairly for professional care. We were very poor. Nina earned enough money for necessities, but there was never a cent left over for treats or entertainment. For those, all we had (and it was enough) were stories of when Mother was a girl, stories told and retold so often over the evenings of our childhood that even today any story can be recalled complete from her random notes written on the back of yellowed prescription blanks or on thin, slippery onionskin papers held firmly together with straight pins.

In Battle Creek, Michigan, in 1898, when Nina was nearing the end of her first full year of college work, the president of the college sent for her.

"Miss Case," he said, "I've been talking to your teachers. We have a Seventh-Day Adventist school in St. Joe, Michigan, which needs a teacher. You are only thirteen years old; you're really much too young to get the most out of your college classes, and you'll be too young to graduate from our two-year course a year from now. We have a rule that no one under sixteen can get a diploma. We've decided that, for your own good, you should take our teacher-training course this summer and teach for a year or two. Then you can come back and get your degree when you will be old enough to appreciate your classes." He was pleased with the arrangement they had all made for Nina's future.

"I don't want to be a teacher," Nina said flatly.

"Well, what do you think you do want to do?" the president asked.

"I want to be a doctor."

"A doctor! That's no field for a woman. Men are doctors. We will talk of this again before the term ends."

Nina, dismissed, went home to Sister Lightner.

I wonder what he meant, Nina said to herself, when he said medicine was no field for women. He acted as though he had made a mistake in talking to me at all.

Some weeks later they did talk again. Sister Lightner was present at the conference between Nina and the president. They both urged her to take advantage of the great opportunity that was being offered, to grow up a bit, to do useful work. School could wait. Then came the clincher.

"The school in St. Joe has only three beginning grades. The children will love you. The school is in a house that also has a small apartment for the teacher."

What thirteen-year-old girl could resist the love of small children and an apartment of her own? Especially a girl who for two years had eaten the bread of charity. By agreeing to go, Nina could give Sister Lightner and little Will a year's free lodging in her very own place. She agreed.

Nina studied teaching methods during the next summer session of the college, and in early September she and Sister Lightner and Will moved into Nina's apartment in St. Joseph, Michigan. Nina started teaching immediately, and by June of the following year, at the close of school, she was almost convinced that teaching should be her life's work. She and the Lightners returned to Battle Creek in midsummer. Nina was prepared to discuss with the president a possible change of curriculum leading to a degree in education, but she was summoned to a conference for a totally different discussion.

"Miss Case," the president began, "how would you like to go to California?"

What a question! Everyone wanted to go to California. By 1899 the railroads had opened the West to ordinary people. If one were lucky enough to have the means, one could go to California, that still-magical never-never land of sun and gold and ripe fruit, without risking one's life. Everyone wanted to go to California.

"We have a school in the northernmost county in California, on the banks of Eureka Bay. There are thirty-two children there who need a teacher."

He spoke of the glowing reports from the parents of the fifteen little children she had been teaching in St. Joe, and the enthusiastic comments of the church elders there. He pointed out that she was still only fourteen years old—plenty of time for college later.

"We would never consider sending a young girl way out there all alone, but if Sister Lightner will go with you, the church will pay for all of you to go."

They went.

They had trouble getting reservations west from Chicago. The Spanish-American War was drawing to a close in Cuba, but the United States had undertaken to quell the insurrection against Spanish rule in the Philippines. Troop trains were going north, south, and west in disorderly spasms. Our little group left, finally, on a tourist sleeper filled with officers and men. The trip from Chicago to San Francisco, always long, was delayed and complicated by the confusion of blocked intersections ahead.

During the long cinder-filled days, Nina entertained little Will with adventure stories she wove out of the passing landscape—stories of pioneers, Indians, rattlesnakes, and buffalo, of evil men who were caught and punished, of good young men and women who always won and never died.

After the first day, two young officers on the seat ahead asked permission to turn their seats around and join in the storytelling. Sister Lightner gave consent, reluctantly. Nina was shy at first, but the obvious enjoyment of her two new listeners reassured her. More and more of the boys joined the group, standing in the aisles, leaning over the backs of the seats, perching on the arms.

Mother told us years later that it became a real strain for her to invent new stories day after day. Scheherazade, threatened by actual death for a thousand and one nights, found the same chore an even greater strain. Nina told us that she would prop herself up on one elbow in her berth at night and plan ahead for the next day's story as she watched the night-quiet, moon-washed landscape slide by outside her window. During the days when the train chugged and smoked its way across the western deserts and when the white alkali dust coming through the open windows drifted over them all, she was ready with a ploy to move one or another of the boys into her story. Joe, Jim, Horace, Steve—each one in turn rode for help on a galloping horse, fought his way out of an impossible and implausible situation, saved the wagon train, captured the bandits. The boys loved being heroes; they slapped each other on the back, they hooted and shouted with glee. The days passed more quickly for all except Sister Lightner, who sat in puzzled disapproval. She felt she was betraying her trust to allow Nina to become the center of so much enthusiastic male attention, but each time she tried to bring the story sessions to a close, she was overruled by the young soldiers.

They said goodbye to each other in San Francisco. Our little group proceeded to Eureka and the boys embarked for the Philippines.

...7

The church school at Eureka, California, was not at all like Nina's previous school in St. Joseph, Michigan. California had proved to be fertile ground for Seventh-Day Adventist missionaries. So many new churches and church schools were being organized there in so many new towns far from each other that the printed materials supplied by Brother Leeland's printing plant in Williamsport, Pennsylvania, had reached only the schools in the San Francisco and Los Angeles areas. Nina's one-room school in Eureka had no supplies at all. There were no books except a few old "worldly" books discarded by the public school. There was not even a blackboard. Nina had been instructed to add the doctrines of the church to her lessons and to delete from the books anything that might undermine the children's faith.

Using only the Bible for the beginners' class, she started with the story of the baby Moses. She sketched the land of Egypt and the river Nile on the floor in the front of the room, telling the children the story of the poor slaves, called Israelites, under the power of the Egyptians. The first week, the beginners learned to sight-read the words Egypt, king, Israelites, Nile River, boy, girl, princess, work, play. They learned to count from one to ten. The words and numbers were written down for them to take home at night. All the children brought Bibles to school after the first day and they learned how to find the place where the story begins. As soon as they learned to recognize and print one set of words, the story would be continued onward. The older children joined the beginners' hour, helping the little ones so as to hurry the story along.

The family of Moses was selected from the entire school. There was Amram, the father of Moses; there was Jochebed, the mother, Aaron, the brother, and Miriam, the sister. Moses himself started as a beginner and grew to be an eighth-grader as the story progressed. The rest of the children were Israelites or Egyptian nobles, soldiers, slave drivers. Everyone had a part as they first read the story, then acted it out. Parents became excited and helped the children at home. Nina added many events not recorded in the Bible. By spring each child could pick up the Bible and read, scarcely stumbling over the words. Parents were amazed at the progress their little ones had made. Ministers of the church visited the school, which became famous in the church as an example of what a church school could do.

The older classes used the worldly books as a foundation. Nina supplemented that material with problems in arithmetic and words for spelling from the Bible, poetry from the Psalms, memory tests from Proverbs.

In the schoolhouse yard on the hill overlooking the town, the children were getting ready, between rain showers, to cross the Red Sea. The play had reached such proportions that it had outgrown the schoolroom and moved outdoors. A stump of a giant redwood tree in the yard, big enough to seat all thirty-two children and their teacher, served usually for an outdoor stage. But that day, a month before the school term was to end, the older children had dug the Red Sea in the yard, heaping the dirt on both sides to represent the held-back waters.

The Israelites gathered on the bank of the Red Sea. Moses, Aaron, and Miriam, with the singers, crossed over first. Moses stood with uplifted rod on the far shore. The singers sang "Onward, Christian Soldiers" lustily as the rest of the Israelites entered the channel. Around the schoolhouse, with wild shrieks and fierce gestures, in all sorts of costumes and carts, came the Egyptians. The crossing was accomplished. The Egyptians lay dead in the channel while the Israelites danced and sang wildly on the other side.

Nina blew her whistle and sent the last child into the schoolhouse. She stood by the Red Sea and laughed. That was a good show! she said to herself. She remembered, she said years later, the acting out of the building of the pyramids. She remembered the court scenes they had played, and remembered "the plagues, which were especially funny." "He that is of a merry heart hath a continual feast."

When she entered the schoolroom, the children had begun to quiet down.

"If you want to start the trip into the desert on Monday, you must all study hard and have perfect lessons. We must reach and settle the Land of Canaan by the time the school year closes. We have many adventures ahead of us in the desert—wild beasts, desert tribes of wild men, snakes, earthquakes, fires, starvation, thirst, and sickness of spirit and body."

The children, wide-eyed with anticipation, settled down to earnest work.

We have an anomaly here. Three years before, Nina was in danger of becoming the "mother of liars" for doing exactly what she was doing now. Then she had been humiliated, reprimanded, and chastised for writing and directing plays. Now she was praised. Then, in tears and rebellion, she had watched the fire curl up and burn her creations. Now, during damp pauses between the drizzles of the northern California rainy season, she laughed with delight at her creations, examples to others of how bricks could be made without straw.

The rainy season continued until late May. The skies were a dull gray that never changed. Rain came down in straight lines, gentle, steady, sometimes stopping only to start again without fanfare. Great green slugs crawled over the boardwalks, the grass, the bushes. Nina longed for the sun, or even for a storm. The damp monotony was smothering. Often after school she would walk down to sit on a high wall by the bay to watch a wood-fed railway engine with its overbig smokestack puff its way over the creaking trestle out into the bay, each dragging car behind loaded with one great redwood log. The logs would be dumped into the bay to float and collect together until the lumber boats came to hoist them aboard and take them to the San Francisco railheads. When the train engineer pulled the lever that let down one side of the freight cars, and when the great logs rolled into the bay, sending up waterspouts of spray and foam, California seemed somewhat less monotonous.

One Sunday she packed a lunch and started to walk to Mt. Shasta. Mt. Shasta turned out to be many more miles away than it had appeared to be from her schoolroom window. Great solitary mountains always loom near. She walked and walked but she succeeded only in losing herself in a redwood forest. Ground water rose alarmingly as the rain began again. She was rescued in the early evening from a patch of high ground by a man in a boat and arrived back in damp, dark, sleeping Eureka in a milk wagon.

One afternoon the wind started to blow and the leaden sky turned black. Nina shepherded the children from the school, all of them leaning against the buffeting winds, to their homes in the town. Soon the great sheets of lightning, the scream of the rising wind, the roar of the thunder over the bay were a welcome change from the persistent quiet drizzle. In the night she was awakened by the wailing of fire sirens, the ringing of church and school bells. She dressed hurriedly and, after reassuring Sister Lightner, ran

out into the street. She had to gasp for breath when the
wind and the rain beat against her face. She followed running townspeople down to the shore, where a lifeboat was
launched repeatedly but each time was washed back to
shore by the pounding surf. In the flashes of lightning she
could see waves breaking mountain-high over a helpless
ship impaled on the rocks of the bar. The ship was a coastal
steamer, the *Wee Ott*, bringing returning Eurekans home
from San Francisco.

A breeches buoy was rigged at last, and those passengers
who would be saved before the ship sank came riding in
through a hell of thundering sound and darkness. Each
survivor who arrived was more frantic than the last.
"Hurry! The ship is filling fast. Hurry!" There was little
time. A flash of lightning illuminated the stern of the ship
as it rose high in the air. The next flash stabbed only at the
wild black empty sea.

After the close of school Sister Lightner, Will, and Nina
left Eureka on a sister ship of the *Wee Ott*. It must have
taken courage to board. Mother was always afraid of water.
They arrived safely in San Francisco and went by train to
San Jose to attend the California Camp Meeting and Conference.

When the Conference closed, Nina was asked to go
throughout the state as a Bible worker for the summer. She
was to organize young people into study groups that would
be more interesting for them than the regular church services on the Sabbath. The idea of Sunday school, already
accepted by the Protestant churches in the East, was new
and untried in the far West.

Sister Lightner's father was ill. She felt she must go to
him. She arranged for Nina to live and travel with Brother
Horace Dayton and his wife while she visited her father in
Pennsylvania. She planned to return in September in time

to take Nina to enroll in the Seventh-Day Adventist
Healdsburg College in Angevin, California, to finish up her
schoolwork. Until then Nina and Brother and Sister Dayton would visit the California churches to organize Sabbath
schools, and at the end of the summer would hold revival
meetings in National City on the Mexican border, a couple
of miles from San Diego.

After the meetings in National City, where large crowds
had come to see the "girl preacher," one of the members of
the San Diego church invited the church workers to spend
a week at his orange ranch outside of town. Nina, pedaling
a borrowed bicycle, returned from the ranch to San Diego
ahead of the Daytons so she could prepare lessons for the
children in the local church for the next day's Sabbath. She
was cutting and pasting cardboard figures when the door
opened and in came Brother Dayton.

Startled, Nina jumped to her feet, spilling the contents
of her lap.

"Oh, you frightened me. I wasn't expecting anyone
home until tomorrow in time for church. Are you all
home? Where are Sister Dayton and Brother and Sister
Walden?" Nina stopped to pick up the pieces of cardboard.

"Here, let me help. I'm sorry I frightened you. I thought
of some things I must do, so I came in tonight. The rest will
be here in the morning," he said.

Nina was uneasy. She didn't like Brother Dayton. She
thought him narrow-minded, selfish, and, in fact, just plain
nosy. Every evening he demanded an accounting of every
moment of the day from everyone. Sister Dayton was meek
under his inquisition, but Nina was often irritated. Perhaps, she thought now, he thinks I might talk to someone
worldly tonight. Silently she gathered her material together to go to her room.

"Please stay. Go on with your work. I really came in

tonight to watch you," he said. "Do you know, Nina, you have beautiful hands. I love to watch you." As he spoke he moved nearer and, removing the cardboard material, took her hands in his. His hands were unpleasantly hot. She pulled free and moved away.

"Don't be offish. I don't believe you've ever had any love or affection. Didn't anyone ever love you or kiss you?"

"No. And I don't want anyone to love me or kiss me." Nina looked at his flushed face. Injun Jake! she thought. A fear ran through her mind. She had been able to forgive Injun Jake because she was fond of him. She was not fond of Brother Dayton. Her muscles tensed and her head drew back as he came over to her.

"You're being very clever, or very stupid, I don't know which," he said. "You know I came in tonight because you are here. You know I'm crazy about you."

She was astonished. "I don't know! I never dreamed of such a thing. You must be out of your mind!" In her surprise and indignation, her alertness to danger relaxed at the wrong time.

He pulled her to him roughly, saying, "You'll never learn any earlier."

With his right hand he caught and held her, twisting her head until her lips were imprisoned against his. His left arm held her right arm against her body, while that hand seized her firm young buttocks and pressed until she was plastered against him.

It would have been smarter if Brother Dayton had used that hand to imprison her left arm. But then, why carp? A sanctimonious, middle-aged churchman of any denomination does not have opportunity for sustained practice in seduction. As any roué will acknowledge, practice does make for more efficiency. Brother Dayton was not efficient. Nina's free hand reached his face and her nails made red welts from his forehead to his chin. He released her abruptly and she escaped behind a table. The door, already ajar, opened wide and Elder Brownell walked in. Elder Brownell was Sister Dayton's father. He stared hard at his son-in-law. Nina, weak from relief, sank down on a chair.

"Well, well, what's going on here?" he asked.

"I had to run in for some notes for my sermon," Brother Dayton said. "I found Nina here. I was just trying to make her see how foolish it is for her to be always tempting me with her attentions."

Nina's astonished "What!" came out louder than she had intended.

"Never mind, Nina," Elder Brownell said kindly. "Don't be alarmed. I was taking my evening walk when I saw Horace come into the house. I thought I might talk to him about family matters, so I followed him in. I've been standing in the hall. I saw and heard everything. This isn't the first time he has made a fool of himself and disgraced his calling." Turning to the humiliated man, he continued, "Let's go out to the ranch. We'll discuss this matter on the way."

It must have been a dreadful evening back at the ranch. "The way of transgressors is hard."

The next Monday morning Elder Brownell accompanied Nina to Angevin, California, site of the Seventh-Day Adventist Healdsburg College. Sister Lightner, whose father had died of his illness, was still in Pennsylvania settling the estate, so Elder Brownell arranged for Nina to live with Elder and Sister Trelour. It was a happy choice. Sister Trelour was a musician almost totally oblivious of any world outside the realm of music. She and Nina were often home alone together, and since Sister Trelour drifted through the real world of housekeeping, religion, and college affairs with detachment and disinterest, their conversations were necessarily confined to music. The hours Mother's children, none of us truly musical, later spent at our piano can be accounted a direct result of Sister Trelour's influence.

Elder Trelour was preoccupied with the college. He was gray, gentle, kindly. He liked to talk with young people. It was to him that Nina went in February when the first school semester was over to consult about her courses for the second half of the college year. Her experience with Brother Dayton had made church work unattractive. The months of study with her peers had reawakened her desire to be a doctor. Elder Trelour was dubious.

"It will take a great deal of money," he said, "and you will have to study for years before you can become a doctor."

"Well, the years will go by just the same," Nina reasoned, "and years from now, if I study medicine, I'll be a doctor. If I go on teaching or doing Bible work, years from now I can only be a teacher or a Bible worker."

"I don't see where you'll get the money to study medicine." Mother remembered how wistful and baffled he seemed to be about money.

"I don't know either," she said, "but there must be a way. I'll find the money somehow."

"You must pray about this," Elder Trelour cautioned. "It would be a shame to spoil a good teacher to make a poor doctor."

It often happens that a deeply felt dream of childhood thwarted, put aside, and neglected for years comes back with renewed enchantment after casual desires have lost their value. Nina was never again to turn away from her childhood ambition. But the medical schools that would admit women were in the East and Nina was in California. By the end of the school year she would need enough money to get from one side of the country to the other. She concentrated her second-semester courses in areas she hoped would be useful for medical school and in June she was given her diploma. That same day she received a letter from Sister Lightner in which a money order sufficient to pay her train fare to Pennsylvania was enclosed. Nina was jubilant.

"If this money hadn't come," she told Elder Trelour, "I would have to stay here and teach to earn a living. Now at least I'll be where the study of medicine is possible! This money is a sign unto me."

Elder Trelour, gentle and baffled, and Sister Trelour, working out intricate harmonics in her head for the final school concert, put her on the train for Pennsylvania.

PART
THREE

*"Some poor fainting, struggling seaman
you may rescue, you may save."*

...1

Nina's trip east to Pennsylvania in 1901 ended in Chicago, where her purse was stolen. Her tickets and the money that had been a sign unto her were gone. The ticket agent to whom she reported her catastrophe took her to the stationmaster. The two men were kind and helpful, but then, why shouldn't they be? Although Nina was now sixteen years old, her hair still hung in neat thick braids down her back. She was tiny—barely five feet tall—slim and shapely. Who wouldn't be kind? Especially in the olden days when a young girl traveling by herself was a phenomenon.

They discovered from her that the Battle Creek Sanitarium had a branch sanitarium in Chicago, the first small doctor-hospital complex to reach out to the sick and the poor in any major American city. Perhaps if they called the hospital, someone would be willing to help her. Battle Creek Sanitarium, the Chicago branch, and the girl were, after all, of the same faith. The stationmaster found the telephone number and talked to the doctor in charge. He was relieved to hear the doctor say, "Keep her right there. My wife and I will come immediately."

Dr. David Paulson and his wife, Mary, took Nina home with them. At supper she told them her dream of studying medicine; she was much less tentative in her mind, she told them, because she really believed the money to come east, where her only possibility of studying medicine lay, was Heaven-sent.

"It will mean a lot of hard work, and a lot of money," Dr. David said.

"Oh, I don't mind hard work. And money? Well, the

Lord has indicated that He will make room for me. And I guess he will."

"Suppose you stay here in Chicago for a while," Dr. David proposed. "We'll see what can be done. Tomorrow we'll see if we can't find some sort of job for you." He arranged for Nina to have a room at the nurses' dormitory at the hospital, and provided her with a meal ticket for the hospital dining room.

She moved into her new room, and at dawn the next morning she dressed and walked quietly outside. She explored the area, frantically trying to imagine what kind of work she could do to earn money. Often a crisis must occur before we learn to face what is real; Nina finally was facing the reality of money. No miracle occurred, and she attended morning worship and went in to breakfast penniless. But at breakfast she asked one of the nurses at her table if there were not some things the hospital was doing that required help other than nursing, for which she was unqualified, or kitchen work.

"There's a printing office where they print *Lifeboat,* a magazine devoted to our work for the prisoners in the state prisons," the nurse offered.

"Where is the press?" Nina asked eagerly.

"Around the corner to the left, in the old annex."

Nina went around the corner and entered the printing plant. The office was small and crowded with desks, supplies, and unsold past issues of the magazine. The sound of the hand presses in the next room was loud. The man in charge of the office explained the purpose of the magazine.

"What's the circulation?" Nina asked.

"Twenty-four thousand copies," he replied, "but we can't keep going much longer unless we raise it to fifty thousand."

"Have you ever tried to sell it on the newsstands, or on the street?"

"No, it's not the sort of magazine people buy on news-stands."

"Give me fifty copies. I'll see if it will sell on the street."

"O.K.," he said, smiling. "You can try. I think you're a little crazy, but you can try."

She left the office with fifty copies of *Lifeboat* on her arm. At the nearest busy corner, she was frightened. The maze of streetcar tracks, the clang of the trolleys, the rumbling of the elevated trains overhead made selling magazines in a big city very different from selling books before Christmas in a small town. She thought of going back to the hospital, then said aloud, "Come now! Do with your might what your hands find to do. Remember?"

"Did you speak?" asked a man passing by.

"Yes. Please buy a *Lifeboat*. It's a magazine devoted to the reform of prisoners. You really will enjoy reading it."

"How much?" he asked, feeling in his pocket.

"Ten cents."

He took the paper and dropped the coin in her hand. One hour later she was back in the *Lifeboat* office, every copy sold. She was beaming and the printer was astonished.

"How much do I owe you for the magazines?"

"One and one-half cents a copy," he replied.

She left the *Lifeboat* office with $4.25 held tightly in her hand. If I can earn this much in one hour, she thought, I can earn real money working an eight-hour day. She began her first eight-hour day the next morning.

Within a week she had organized the women of the local church into a sales force. She trained them mercilessly.

"Don't be lazy. Put in honest time. Decide how many hours a day you can give to the work, then keep on working until that number of hours is finished. If you don't sell, don't worry. If you put in the time, you'll begin to sell, sooner or later. Sell door to door but sell to everyone you meet. There's no way to tell by a person's appearance whether he'll buy or not. Try everyone."

She didn't exactly tell the women that there's a sucker born every minute, but in a few weeks, following her instructions, the women were selling all over Chicago. By charging them two cents a copy, Nina made fifty cents on every hundred copies they sold. The women donated their profits to the work of the church. Nina kept hers. In the fall she enrolled in night classes at Atheneum College. She sold magazines eight hours a day during the long, cold, dark winter and studied German and chemistry at night. She was wonderfully happy to be on a straight path to her goal.

...2

Late in the next summer Nina acquired an unexpected assistant. Marie was a Swedish girl from Minnesota, twenty-two years old, an orphan, raised in a county home until she was twelve. From then on she had worked for her keep for various farm families. When she was eighteen she began to receive three dollars a month in wages. Her education had been sporadic and scanty—she could read and write, possibly well enough to pass a fifth-grade examination.

Somewhere in her life she had decided to become a trained nurse. She saved every cent she earned, going out at night when she could, after a long day's work, to help someone clean house or to mind children for extra money. She had come to Chicago to start nurse's training, unaware of the necessity of a minimum formal education to enter the school. She arrived at the Chicago Sanitarium early one morning and asked to see the "head doctor."

"The doctor's not here this morning," his secretary said.

"Do you have an appointment?"

"No, but I must see him."

"Are you sick?"

"No, ma'am, I ain't sick. I just got to see the head doctor. I can wait."

And there she waited all morning and through the noon hour. Nurses and attendants went by the door to get a glimpse of her as word was passed along about her strange appearance. She was tall and awkward-looking, with thick, dirty blond hair piled high on her head, straggling locks hanging down on every side about her tanned, freckled face. She had no hat; her shirtwaist and skirt were not together at the waist; she wore boys' heavy work shoes over bare feet. All her belongings were tied up in an old Paisley shawl that she kept close to her.

When Nina came in after one o'clock, a little late for dinner, one of the nurses said, "Go look at the freak waiting for Dr. David in the parlor. She's prehistoric!"

"Is she sick?" Nina asked.

"No, she says not. She just says, 'I got to see the head doctor.' " The nurse sneered. "She won't tell anyone what she wants."

"Well, why should she? If she wants to see the doctor, that's her business. Sometimes it's important to speak to an exact person," Nina said indignantly.

"I guess you're right. It's just that she looks so funny, no one can imagine where she came from or what she wants."

"Maybe we look funny to her." Nina was softened by the nurse's apologetic tone. "How long has she been here? Has she had any dinner?"

"I don't know. I guess not. She came about eight o'clock and hasn't budged since."

Nina crossed the hall and went in. Marie was dozing. Nina had a moment to notice her work-worn hands with broken nails, her chapped wrists, her bruised ankles. She shook Marie gently.

"Excuse me, but have you had any dinner?"

Marie was embarrassed at having fallen asleep. "No, but I'm all right."

"Won't you please come and eat with me? I'm late for dinner, too. Dr. David won't be in until three o'clock. We've lots of time." Marie looked anxiously at her bundle. "Your things will be safe here; no one will touch them."

Marie stood up. She was even taller and more ungainly standing than sitting. "I ain't fit to go to table. I was on the train all the whole night," she said, looking at her hands.

"We'll go to the washroom first. While you're washing, I'll go tell the cook to give us something for dinner." She was gone and back again at the lavatory before Marie was ready.

While they were eating, Nina found that farm people were not so very different from mountain people. By the time they had finished, Nina knew a great deal more about Marie than Marie had meant to tell. Nina's tender heart ached as Marie's story unfolded. Fed and with a friend, Marie lost her dogged, stolid façade and showed spirit and hopefulness.

"I tell you what," Nina said. "I'll see Dr. David first. I can get him to see you." While Marie waited again in Dr. David's parlor, Nina went into his office and explained the situation.

"You've probably told Marie's story better than she could," Dr. David sighed, "but what can we do with her? She certainly can't enter training."

"She can stay with me in my room. I'll find work for her. She can go to adult education classes at night until she's ready for training. Oh, Dr. David, please see her. You'll realize right away that she's a real person."

Marie was called in. She was told that the road to nursing was long and hard. It meant years of hard work and study. She would first have to complete the equivalent of a high school education; she would have to work so that, as soon as possible, she could pay for her board and room; and she would have to clothe herself. All this had to be done before she could join the nurses' class.

"That's all right, Doc," Marie said. "I'll work for twenty years to be a nurse. You won't never lose nothin' on me."

"All right, then," Dr. David agreed. "Nina, I'm holding you responsible for her."

"I'll be responsible." Nina stood up. "I'll be more than responsible. I'll be happy. We can help each other. It will be wonderful."

Marie, towering over Nina, bent down and put her big, rough hand gently on Nina's shoulder. They looked at each other for a moment, both smiling, then turned and went out together.

In her room, carefully and with the tact she had learned in the mountains, Nina began to pull Marie together. The blouse and skirt could not be pulled together, but Marie's hair, washed and combed, turned out to be a dark-gold cloud, the color of ripe wheat. They subdued the cloud into a thick, neat bronze chignon. The wayward tendrils that still escaped were snipped short so that random curls softened the magnificent bone structure of Marie's rugged face. The next morning they bought Marie a green dress that complimented her statuesque proportions and emphasized her narrow, bright-green eyes. They bought stockings and shoes and a hat. It's odd to remember that in those days hats were as necessary for outdoor wear as shoes for women of any class.

The next day they went out to sell *Lifeboat.* Nina chose a quiet neighborhood, and for the first dozen houses she did the talking while Marie observed in the background. Then Nina took the opposite side of the street and let Marie try alone. Poor Marie, shy and awkward, sold nothing all day. She was not discouraged; she was willing to try again and again. Three days later she started to sell, and the worst was over. They soon took different routes. Marie started out every day at eight o'clock and worked until four. Every night she counted her money with wonder and delight. She paid back the loan from Nina for her clothes. She enrolled in night adult education classes shortly after Nina enrolled in Atheneum College. They studied together in the night, Marie puzzling over her lessons long after Nina was asleep.

Marie lost the tan and the freckles that in those days were considered unattractive. Her beautiful hair, her bright narrow eyes, and her straight, beautiful stride caused heads to turn as she walked by. She was on her way.

...3

"Has Marie come home yet? Any letters for me?" Nina asked at the hospital desk on her way from night school to her room on the top floor.

"One," replied the clerk. He shuffled through a stack of letters until he found one for her. "No, Marie's not home yet."

She was surprised to see that the letter was from Dr. David Paulson. She had seen him at supper in the hospital dining room and he had said nothing about writing to her. This, she thought, must be something very important. She sat down on the arm of a nearby chair and opened the envelope.

Dear Miss Case,

How would you like to represent the *Lifeboat* magazine and the Sanitarium Idea at the Southern Camp Meetings this summer? We will send a nurse in uniform with you as chaperon and helper. You will take orders for *Lifeboat*, get subscriptions of money for our enterprises, viz: prison work, Sunday jail services in police stations, and for our Rescue Home. If the venture succeeds, we will see that you have money to enter medical school in the fall, providing the Conference Committee agrees.

On this trip you will have transportation, room and board, and a percentage on all magazine subscriptions you sell. We will outfit you with uniform and necessary baggage.

Come in tomorrow and we will talk it over. In the meantime, pray for light and guidance. It will be a great responsibility for one so young. We cannot give you a set program. You will have to decide how to make this work, but from what we have observed, you will be able to do this if you keep your humble, God-fearing spirit.

> Sincerely,
> DAVID PAULSON, M.D.

Nina gave a shout of joy and danced around the deserted hospital lobby waving her letter and chanting, "He's made room! He's made room! I knew it could be, and now He's made room!"

The desk clerk was agog. "What's happened? What is it? Did someone leave you a fortune?"

"No. Better than that! The Lord has made room for me!"

She sped up the stairway to her room, where behind a closed door she could soberly and devoutly thank Him from the depths of her innocent heart.

Weeks of planning and preparation followed. It was decided that Nina and Mrs. Hale, the nurse, would spend one week at each of the Southern Summer Camp Meetings. They would sell *Lifeboat* in the nearby towns, and Nina would speak twice at each encampment, once in an afternoon service on the Sanitarium Idea and once in the evening meeting in the big tent on the plight of prisoners and the church's need for money to bring them hope, medical supplies, and, where possible, a new attitude toward themselves and their lives. The printing plant worked night and day to print and then to mail thousands of copies of the magazine to the post offices in every city where they were scheduled to stop.

Nina arranged for Marie to take over her entire magazine operation in Chicago. Marie was delighted to be put in charge of the church women and to reap half a cent a copy of unearned income. She was not yet in training, but five years later she would graduate at the head of her nursing class. Nobody never lost nothin' on her.

On the fifth of May, Nina and Mrs. Hale were ready to leave on their tour. The nurse, a beautiful, stately, white-haired woman, wore a white uniform with a navy-blue cap and shoulder-length pleated veil edged with white piqué. Nina wore a sheer navy-blue cotton voile uniform with narrow white collar and cuffs, and a nurse's cap of navy blue, with a sheer veil down to her shoulders in back. They must have made a striking pair—Nina with her long dark braids and her clear light-blue eyes, the nurse surrounded by that aura of competence and rectitude that every mature nurse carries with her.

Wherever they were, on the train, in the depot, on the street, they sold *Lifeboat.* They would take a bundle of magazines from their luggage and in no time at all it was gone. In cities where they stopped for the Camp Meeting week, the post office was their first port of call. They sold from the post office on through the town, inviting everyone they met to come to the meetings held on the campgrounds. By the time Nina's scheduled speeches were to be made late in the week, the big tent was full. There was not, you must realize, a great deal to do in the evenings in those days. And the impact of our two women, saintly youth joined with white-haired competence, drew crowds. They progressed in increasing triumph from Little Rock to Memphis to Nashville, where Nina, who was the Camp Meeting authority on prisons, visited her first penitentiary; to New Orleans, Baton Rouge, Jackson, Montgomery, Birmingham, and Atlanta.

As they progressed from city to city, invitations came for Nina to speak in other churches and for other organizations; the WCTU, the Anti-Saloon League, various local prison-reform groups that knew a great deal more about the appalling state of the prisons than Nina knew. Soon there was no time to sell *Lifeboat.* At that point Nina conceived a brilliant idea. She decided to sell subscription blocks, one hundred subscriptions minimum. The churches and groups buying the subscriptions would know that the money they paid would be used for help for the prisoners, and the magazines would not go to the subscribers but to the prisoners. What a great idea! The persons who gave the money for good work would not be burdened with the bad conscience that results from throwing away unread uplift material, and the prisoners might very well benefit. Then or now, there has never been enough to do in prison. It is very possible that a young offender would be strengthened to change himself as he read how someone older and more fatally trapped in a circle of criminal activities had begun a new life, substituting new habits for those that led him inevitably into repeated prison terms.

Thousands of subscriptions poured in. In that one summer the circulation of *Lifeboat* increased from 24,000 to 75,000.

Nina's speech for the afternoon services was simple and direct. She spoke first on the general Sanitarium Idea, the program in the Seventh-Day Adventist sanitarium for treating the whole patient with a nourishing nonharmful diet, with trusted medicines, with trained nursing care, with hope, and with confidence in God. She spoke of the medical missionary work of the Chicago branch of Battle Creek Sanitarium. She described the trips she had taken with the visiting nurses to the district called "back of the yards" in Chicago; the almost hopeless task, for this handful of workers, of reaching out to the desperately poor, desperately ignorant, sick, and bewildered people of the area.

Then she talked about the home treatment of simple diseases. Mrs. Hale, the nurse, gave the treatments on a cot on the platform, selecting a patient from the audience. Nina explained how to treat a cold, toothache, sleeplessness, headache, earache, stomachache, boils, backache, frozen feet, sprains, and tantrums thrown by both children and those well past childhood. It must have been an enjoyable show.

Then she gave a simple talk about diet. She talked about the nutritive value of whole-grain cereal, honey, fruit, vegetables, and berries. She told about the fine protein value of nuts, milk, and beans. And she extolled the thirst-quenching virtue and the medical benefit of pure, cold water. With St. Francis of Assisi, she praised "Sister Water, who is useful, humble, precious, and pure." Poor Sister Water in these latter inattentive and uncaring days! Without her, so useful, precious, and pure, what will become of us all?

She spoke about the bad effects of liquor, tobacco, hate,

bad temper, selfishness, and envy on the health of the human body. Since she didn't drink or smoke, hated no one, was sweet-tempered and unselfish, and had never known the corrosive physical and psychological effects of envy, she must have been convincing. One gray-haired farmer in Tennessee came up after one meeting and put twenty-five dollars in Nina's hand.

"Here," he said. "This is my next year's tobacco money. I'm through chewin'. Use this to help one of them poor folk in the big city that's got it so bad."

The evening service was more emotional. The best preachers, the best hymns, the best music, the highest pitch of emotion were the goals. Nina spoke midway in the service. She had to keep her talk simple and somewhat vague. Her association with prisons, prisoners, police stations, and criminals reformed or unreformed was nonexistent. But she had good material to work with. From my research I am impressed with the imaginative vigor of that church in its dedication to the alleviation of the appalling plight of prisoners. In those days almost nobody else cared. She must have been given firsthand accounts, because I have found firsthand accounts, in books my mother never read, which echo my childhood memories of her prison stories. As she spoke more often, she gained in power both to enthrall and to convince.

About the Rescue Home she had firsthand information. This old-time halfway house took in any lost soul who came, but the bulk of its residents were runaway teenage girls. Nina had gone there frequently, not just because she liked children and was concerned especially with these bedraggled, forlorn, and hostile little girls, but also because she felt they could usefully spend their time making special treats for the little ones confined in the hospital over birthdays and holidays. As they worked together in groups,

Nina heard their stories and understood their attitudes; and she grieved for them. She must have been effective in her talks about the Rescue Home, because, for instance, the mayor of Amory, Mississippi, who had been at the evening service and had already contributed generously, came to the railroad station the next morning as Nina and Mrs. Hale were boarding their train. He drew Nina aside and pressed a hundred-dollar bill into her hand.

"Use this for the Rescue Home. Our only daughter ran away many years ago. We have never heard from her. Help some young girl now for her sake. And for ours." His walk, as he turned away, was rigid with sorrow.

Toward the end of the summer tour, a leader of the Women's Christian Temperance Union heard Nina speak. A few days later a letter came from the WCTU central office asking Nina to join a lecture tour throughout the United States. She was offered all expenses and $200 a month. Even with her newfound respect for money, she wasn't tempted. She tucked the letter away to use as a reason to consult with the Conference Committee about her future.

When she returned to Chicago she was greeted with enthusiasm and acclaim. The sanitarium staff was overjoyed with the money and pledges that were pouring in. All their projects had taken on new vigor. Nina was in demand everywhere to tell about the trip and her work. She was busy, but not so busy as to forget to ask for a meeting with Elder Allen, the chairman of the Conference Committee.

She opened the meeting with him by producing the letter from the WCTU. He was impressed by the salary, which was indeed a large one for those days. He asked Nina what she thought about joining the Temperance Union tour.

"I couldn't," she said. "I want to be a doctor, and now

is the time to start."

Elder Allan was silent. Dr. David Paulson had explained Nina's desire to him, but the elder had put off facing what was, to him, a doubtful and dangerous idea. But the cards were on the table now. He tried to explain his reluctance to give approval to such a project.

"You see, Nina, it's such a risk. Worldly schools, especially medical schools, are full of atheists. It would be a hard task for you to go to a worldly medical school like that and still keep your faith. We have lost almost all of our young men who have tried it. They're now out of the church and work in worldly hospitals. Of the few who have returned to our institutions, many of these have brought worldly ideas and practices into our hospitals." Then, seeing the cloud of disappointment on her face, he added, "We'll pray about it. I'll call the Conference Committee together. I'll talk to Dr. Kellogg at Battle Creek. If the way opens up for you to go and still keep your hold on the Truth, we will help you."

Dr. John Harvey Kellogg was the director of the Battle Creek Sanitarium, the most successful of the hospitals under Seventh-Day Adventist control. As director, Dr. Kellogg was so important to the church that he was consulted on every problem in the Midwest area.

With what reassurance she could find in Elder Allen's statements, Nina had to hold her peace and wait.

A week later she was invited to speak at an afternoon meeting of the entire staff of Battle Creek Sanitarium in Battle Creek, Michigan, and she was invited to a supper at the home of Dr. Kellogg after the meeting. This day happened to be, by coincidence, her eighteenth birthday. She spoke well and was enthusiastically received by the staff, and at supper she met W. W. Kellogg, the doctor's brother, who was somewhat tense and apprehensive about a new business he was about to begin. Little did Nina know at supper that night that the idea of corn flakes and shredded wheat was on the verge of being revealed to a cooked-cereal world.

Two weeks later, Elder Allen called Nina into his office in Chicago. He was abrupt.

"The Conference Committee has met. The only way the church could give approval to your idea of being a doctor or could justify spending the amount of money it would take to see you through to the actual practice of medicine would be if you would marry one of our preachers."

This was a bombshell.

"Marry!" Nina was stunned. "Marry! I don't understand."

"You could study medicine in the winter, and work with our preacher in the summers in church work. There would be less danger of your being weaned away from your religion. You must realize, Nina, that it is our responsibility, and our deepest concern, to save your immortal soul."

"I can't just marry anyone! I've never even thought of marriage."

"Now, don't be hasty. We mean married for the sake of the church, not married in a worldly sense."

He went on to explain that in these "last days" men and women who were getting ready for "translation" were above the earthly idea of marriage, that a woe had been pronounced on all of God's people who had children in the last days.

"If you agree to this," he argued, "you can go on and study medicine with a free mind."

"Do you have anyone in mind that I should marry?" Nina asked. She was trying to make this extraordinary proposition seem real.

"No. We have several in mind, but we've made no decision. You can, however, start medical school now. As soon as we've found the right one, we'll let you know."

"Must I decide now?"

"I don't see why not. There's nothing to discuss. Either you agree, or we must start thinking about what other work you can do."

Nina stared out of the window. The unreality of the discussion made her slow-witted. A giant black crow flapped down to perch on the slenderest topmost branch of a yew hedge outside the window. He teetered perilously until he was sure the spray of yew would hold his weight. At rest, his feathers iridescent purple in the afternoon sunlight, the crow surveyed the garden. Nina wrenched her mind away from this normal oddity of nature.

"Very well," she said. "Do what you think best."

Elder Allen was unaccountably uneasy. "If I were you, I would say nothing to anyone about this arrangement, especially not to Dr. David or Dr. Kellogg. I must ask you to promise me that."

Nina agreed. She left the office and walked home, as she said later, on leaden feet. The girl who had danced for joy around a cold, deserted hospital lobby such a short while ago walked back to the same hospital lobby weighed down by a heavy burden of bewilderment and apprehension.

Is it any wonder that I judge my mother to have been panther-prone? Away she went up a road where she knew a panther might lie in wait, else why the leaden feet? What decision should she have made? Her grain-of-mustard-seed faith had moved too many mountains for her to turn back now. She had long trusted authority, even though it had led her into hardship and danger and deprivation. Could she now have rebelled? Maybe she would have agreed to marry the Devil himself rather than lose her heart's desire. But the secrecy demanded of her should have warned her that

there was something not quite right here, something not
exactly acceptable.

Why the secrecy? What went on in the Conference Committee discussion? Who proposed such a compromise between those for and those against? If means to an end must
be hidden with unease and shamefacedness, can those who
demand secrecy complain if the end is not to their liking?
"Say ye to the righteous, that it shall be well with him: for
they shall eat the fruit of their doings."

Nina went to Northwestern Medical School the next day
to enroll. In the rush and hurry of choosing her courses,
finding a room in a convenient boardinghouse, packing and
moving and saying goodbye to the past and welcome to the
future, her spirits rose. What healthy, single-minded girl
can dwell overlong on future dangers? Even panthers tire
of waiting and may drift away.

PART
FOUR

*"I walked in the garden alone,
while the dew was still on the roses."*

...1

Seven young women entered the freshman class of the Northwestern Medical School in 1903. Of the seven, only two were to complete the course and become doctors. Accredited medical schools were just beginning to admit women, and prejudice against them among the faculty and male students was an almost tangible obstacle. They were ridiculed and made the butt of jokes. Male students would line up along both sides of the stairways leading to upstairs classrooms. As the "hen medics" ran the gauntlet, the men made obscene jokes and absurd kissing noises, accompanied by drawn-out m-m-m-ms. It is a recognized fact, even today, that no group is so tasteless and physical in its jokes as young male medical students. For young women who had never heard such language before, it must have been extremely difficult. If one of the women students entered a classroom after the men had assembled, the men would stamp along with every step she took, and they would rise and sit down with her with a loud bump that shook the amphitheater. In a world where a woman who allowed her ankles to be seen below her skirts was called daring, to have the noise her bottom didn't make sitting down on a wooden stool echo through a public hall must have been embarrassing.

But the real discouragement came, Dr. Nina's notes record, from the attitude of the all-male faculty. The professors never called upon women students in the classes. If one of the women insisted on speaking, uncalled upon, no one listened. When students were assigned to local professional or charitable clinics for practical experience to supplement their theoretical classwork, the assignments went to the men. What became the hardest trial for the morale of the women students was the tacit encouragement by the professors of harassment by male students—the half-hidden smile, the busy paperwork just at the time when discipline firmly applied could have brought order. The women had a hard row to hoe.

Of the five who didn't make it, one in particular was interesting. She affected a mannish style in her dress and in her short-cropped hair. This was not an unusual affectation in women medical students. But the girl was a true eccentric. Nothing about the human body, male or female, dismayed her. She tried out the three-legged stools in each classroom the first week of classes and pasted on the underside of a stool in each room her own name written in clear, large letters. So she laid claim to "her" stool, one that seemed to fit best the contours of her spare anatomy. When she entered a classroom, late or early, she found her stool, and if someone was sitting on it, she dumped him off. She conceived a passion, early on, for kidneys, and in her second year was asked by the administration to leave for "insubordination and impertinence" for a continuing battle with one of the professors over the diagnosis and treatment of kidney diseases, a battle she even took to the local press. She may have been in the right; medical science advances by small steps through those who question established ideas. She may have been merely an eccentric. We'll never know.

The two who did make it through to a medical degree were Nina Case and Stella Harmon. They met in the first week of school and, since both were limited in money for living expenses, immediately moved together to a boardinghouse room near the school. I expect each one separately would have made it on her own, but it surely did neither any harm to face that hostile world together. Stella was a splendid girl—calm, intelligent, hard-working, well adjusted, tolerant, and totally disinterested in religion. Nina was at once ecstatic about being where she had so longed to be and sharply defensive about being influenced in any way in her religious life. This new world was, for her, peopled by a different race than any she had known since she left her father. To her, all people outside the church were poor misguided souls who, if they did not see and accept the light, would be destroyed and lost forever. To her, what the Lord and the church thought of her was all that mattered. To Stella, what the Lord and the church thought of anybody or anything was of no concern whatsoever. So they could live together, working out their small human everyday problems and helping each other in their studies without either one being a threat to the other. The lectures and the new things Nina was learning sometimes made her wonder and have doubts, but Stella did not make her uneasy.

Perhaps the reason was that their relationship, though warm, was superficial. Nina had been living for years in a world dominated by an esoteric religious philosophy of which Stella knew nothing. Nina had been warned that association with worldly people would undermine her faith. Lasting friendships evolve from candid revelations of self from one person to another, but Nina, protecting her inner life from intrusion, made Stella an outsider and made the relationship between them ephemeral. When their ways were to part, the girls were to separate forever. Stella was never to reappear in Nina's life except as a pleasant, vaguely defined memory.

But in their two years of medical school together, Nina and Stella complemented each other in their work. Nina's mind could grasp everything she learned and translate it into simple, logical language; she never had to cram for examinations because she had only to imagine that she was explaining to simple mountain people what she knew to find fixed in her memory everything she'd studied. Stella, who had grown up in a doctor's family, found all the complicated medical language familiar. Nina would explain to Stella what they had learned, and Stella would drill them both in the medical terminology for what they had learned. They passed all their examinations with ease.

Although Nina was to tell us stories later about her years in medical school, in all the boxes of notes I found only one description of an actual class. That class was anatomy. This is not surprising. The dissection of a dead human body is a milestone in every medical student's education. More than a milestone. The experience is basic training in the objectivity a doctor must learn in order to discipline empathy.

The anatomy laboratory was on the fifth floor of the college. Stella and Nina, the first students to arrive for the first class, looked in through the glass window of the door. The stone-topped tables were bare. As the two girls, scalpels and forceps in hand, pushed open the swinging door, a rush of such foul air surrounded them that they struggled to keep from gagging.

"How terrible!" Nina said. "Did you ever smell anything worse?"

"My father says one's sense of smell quickly gets hardened to anything." Stella held a handkerchief to her nose.

"Well, we'll smell it for six weeks. I hope he's right."

Nina walked down the room, trying to imagine how she could bring herself to dissect a human body. A gruff voice said, "Heads up!" as one of the janitors came from behind her with a body, arms and legs dangling over his shoulder. "Look out," another man said as she stepped back and stumbled over a body he was dragging by one arm. The bodies were wrapped in preservative-soaked gauze strips. The odor became stronger and the formaldehyde stung her nostrils. She went back to stand beside Stella at the door.

"Isn't it awful?" she asked. "How will we manage?"

"Pull yourself together, kid. Don't you dare let on that anything makes you sick. You'll let yourself in for a lot of jokes. We have to do this, so buck up. Let's be nonchalant."

Nina looked at Stella's pinched, white face and started to laugh.

"Oh, Stella! You don't look a bit nonchalant!"

They were both laughing when the first rush of male students came through the door. The men must have been disappointed that the girls were not incapacitated by their delicate sensibilities. How pleasant it is to contemplate the frustration of petty tormentors! The students were busy for the next half hour finding lockers and choosing bodies. There was one cadaver for each pair of students. The two girls chose a body on the table nearest the door so that when the session was over, they could be the first to leave.

Dissection began with the legs of the cadaver. Nina and Stella worked their way around their table and their body, one reading while the other worked, taking turns. Sometime during each day the professor in charge would stop at one table, and then another, taking up a dissected part with his long forceps and quizzing the dissectors about it. A gallery of students from other tables crowded around to listen and to learn. Nina mentioned in her notes that just once in the six-week session, he stopped at the hen-medic table. His stop was brief and his examination was cursory, but it was handsome of him, in that era, to stop at all. But then, even in those olden days, years of honorable recognition often made older men courtly.

...2

Nina was well into the second semester of her freshman year of medical school when, in April of 1904, a letter came to her from the Illinois Conference of the Seventh-Day Adventist Church. The letter was signed by Elder Allen, Chairman. He was pleased to inform her that the Conference had found the right man for her to marry. His name was Charles Victor Baierle, he was thirty-seven years old, and he was an ordained minister whose current assignment was the formation of new churches in communities heretofore unvisited by church missionaries. The Reverend Mr. Baierle would notify her of the day of his arrival. He would have only one day to spend in Chicago. The minister of the nearest Chicago church had been alerted to hold himself free to perform the marriage ceremony at Charles Baierle's convenience.

Nina said, years later, that Elder Allen's letter came as a psychic shock. Engrossed as she was in what she was doing, she had removed from her mind her promise to marry for the salvation of her soul. She hadn't forgotten; she had put aside her part of the agreement the way we all pack up inconvenient problems of the past, expecting them to sleep their lives quietly away. But the past never stays quiet for long. It confronts us at unguarded moments, demanding recognition, reconciliation.

The Reverend Charles Baierle arrived in Chicago, and he and Nina met in the early morning in the boardinghouse parlor before Nina left for her classes. It was arranged that they would marry in the late afternoon. Each was reassured by the appearance of the other. The Reverend Charles was a small man with a head just slightly too large for his body;

but he was handsome. His hair was dark and wavy, his brown eyes were large and soft. His voice was strikingly melodious. His attitude was gravely impersonal, but he seemed courteous and kind. Nina, her braids gone now, her hair piled neatly on her head, seemed older than her nineteen years. She was nervous and shy, a suitable state of mind, in the eyes of the Reverend, for a young female.

Nina went on to her classes. In the course of the day, two conversations took place. There are notes about them and years later she recounted both conversations to us, her children, in one of our evening story hours. One of the conversations was with a junior-year medical student named Bert Roselle. Nina had rushed down the staircase from her last class and, zipping around the corner to the main corridor, had run full tilt into Bert Roselle, knocking him down.

"What's the hurry? Why the blind rush?" Bert asked as Nina helped him dust himself off and collect his scattered papers. "Do you always shoot down steps and around corners like that?"

"I'm really sorry. Do you think you're hurt?"

"I'm not hurt, except for my vanity. Why the hurry?"

"I'm to be married in two hours to someone I met for the first time today. I'll never get home in time to dress unless I run." Nina started on down the hall.

"Wait! Did you say married? My God, girl, you can't marry someone you've just met!"

Nina hesitated and turned back.

"Wait!"

But Nina shook her head and rushed on.

Stella was in their boardinghouse room when Nina arrived. "I can't believe you mean to go through with this crazy marriage!" she said as Nina was shedding her clothes.

"Stella, please believe me. I have to do it. There's no other way."

"There must be another way. You can't marry an old man."

"I'm only keeping a bargain. I promised if I could study medicine, I'd marry one of their preachers. So they let me study medicine. Besides, he's not an old man. He's thirty-seven."

"That's old! Too old for you. And why is this happening now? Why not before? Why not after you finish school?"

"They didn't have anyone before. Now they've found one."

"But why do you have to marry at all?"

"You wouldn't understand."

"Do you? Do you understand?" Stella was almost shouting.

"I don't know. I really don't know if I understand or not." Nina's bewildered tone made Stella contrite.

"Don't let me upset you, Nina. It's just that when you say you are to marry one of their preachers, it sounds as though it doesn't matter whom you marry as long as it's some preacher or other."

"Well, it doesn't really," Nina explained, "because we are only being married in the church so we can work together in church work, not being married as the world thinks of it."

"It sure sounds queer to me," Stella said.

"So it does to me, now." Nina went into the bath to prepare herself for her wedding.

Seventeen years later, on a dark early-winter evening, Nina would tell her three little children about her wedding day. Now, more than half a century later, time seems to fracture into separate layers the way a single ray of light beamed through a prism scatters into separate colors. I am surprised that the words of a Bert Roselle, a young man who was never to appear in Nina's life again, could come down through all the years between. Do we become immortal by accident? And I'm interested that Stella, walled off so firmly from Nina's inner life as to become a cardboard character, actually was real enough to push against the barriers to help a friend.

When Nina was telling her three little girls about her wedding day, we were in the front room of a second-floor apartment. To save money, no lights burned. A bright coal fire glowed and flickered in a tiny fireplace. Dark shadows moved as the coals sparked and shifted in the grate.

"Maybe I should have listened to Bert Roselle and Stella," Nina said, "but I was too inexperienced. I'd always had to work too hard to know what other adolescents learn at the normal time. There is a big gap in my life I can never fill with experiences I should have had then." She turned her gaze intently on each one of us in turn. "Sometimes I'm afraid. I'm afraid that when you children are older, I won't be able to help you because I won't understand, even then, the things you will already know."

She was talking to herself, of course, but we were listening to her emotions. It is a terrible thing for small children to hear their mother admit that she is afraid. Our mother was the only bulwark we had against the dark of the outside world. We couldn't allow her to be afraid. We urged her not to worry. We assured her passionately that we would never become mysterious, we would always remain understandable. Nina laughed, the fire burned brighter, the shadows were only shadows.

Nina and the Reverend Charles Baierle were married at five o'clock in the afternoon. During the cab ride back to the boardinghouse, it was arranged that Charles would pick up Nina after her last exam at the close of school and they would proceed together by train to the Camp Meeting site outside of Pittsburgh, Pennsylvania. They shook hands cordially at the boardinghouse door and Charles left in the same cab to be on his way to wherever he was going.

...3

Nina and Charles Baierle spent their first night together on a train going from Chicago to Pittsburgh. They had met at the station and had had supper together in the cafeteria before boarding the evening train. I don't know what kind of relationship she had expected would evolve that night; she never said. The accounts I find in her notes of that whole summer are meager and they carry overtones of dissatisfaction and dismay. On the train they talked for a while until the porter came to make up their berths. Charles climbed into the upper berth and went to sleep. Nina lay awake all night. The rhythmic clicking of the wheels kept repeating, "Now you've done it! Now you've done it!" To argue back that she'd done only what she'd promised to do drove away sleep.

Perhaps she had hoped for friendship. Both of them, Charles and Nina herself, knew that their relationship was not to be "worldly." But perhaps she had expected they would be friends. All the next day on the train Charles remained impersonal and preoccupied. When they arrived in Pittsburgh, Charles hired a conveyance to take them and their luggage to the Camp Meeting grounds between Pittsburgh and Union City. They arrived at the reception tent as strange to each other as when they left Chicago.

Some of the elders in charge of the large Camp Meeting were in the reception tent and Nina was introduced for the first time as Mrs. Baierle. They all shook hands and went together to the dining tent for the evening meal. Many more families had come than had been expected, so there was no tent available to accommodate Nina and Charles. The elders helped them carry their baggage to a boarding-house near the grounds. Nina was exhausted from a sleep-less night and a disappointing day. Charles suggested that she rest while he attended the evening camp services. When he had gone, she crawled into bed and didn't awake until Charles had come back and left again for the morning service. He had slept on the other side of the double bed.

Later that day, a horse and wagon took them and the gear necessary for Charles's missionary work to the small town of McKeesport. There they were met by the organist and the Bible worker assigned to Charles for the summer's work. Together they set up the tent, the board benches, the rickety platform, the pulpit, and the organ. There were two chairs for the platform and three gasoline flare lamps, two for light inside the tent and one for outside to illumi-nate the entrance flaps. The tent had a sawdust floor, giving it a fresh, woodsy aroma. They began their meetings im-mediately.

At their first meetings, they sang to empty benches. The Reverend Charles then prayed very loudly so that people on porches of houses near the empty lot they had appro-priated could hear him. Then they all sang another hymn. Charles preached his sermon just inside the opening of the tent; his resonant voice carried far and wide. Gradually, people began to drift in. Before the first week was gone, the tent was full every night. After the last worshiper had left, the benches were stacked against the wall and four army cots were set up in the middle of the tent. There they all slept.

Nina's job was to greet people, telling them how glad the tent company was to see them. She gave out programs, and at the close of the service she gave out tracts to take home.

In the afternoons she organized children's meetings. The thing she stressed to us later about that summer was that she enjoyed the children, and their parents often brought wonderful things to eat to the tent. I can safely surmise that the collections were scant and the missionary group was often hungry.

Nina had an additional and more subtle assignment. Emotional young women and, indeed, not-so-young spinsters would have a personal, almost romantic reaction to Charles's ministry. After most of the worshipers had left, these women would dawdle around, each determined to outwait the others, to have a private moment with the handsome pastor. Nina would join Charles and he would introduce his wife. The women found pressing reasons to leave immediately. So she served a useful purpose; husbands trusted Charles more and women bothered him less.

No wonder she was dissatisfied with that summer. After her triumphal Southern Camp Meeting tour not so long before, when she had been the featured and acclaimed speaker not only to her own fellow churchmen but also to other large and vigorous social-reform groups, when she had met the challenge of raising a large amount of money, when every day had brought new skills and new successes, the whole summer must have been deadly dull for her.

More than dull. Disturbing. In her notes she mentions that the church's approach to recruiting new members in new areas was, in those days, devious. In all their posters, flyers, and announcements, not one indication was given that the missionary workers were Seventh-Day Adventists. Always they were holding "evangelistic meetings" and "Bible study" in a "gospel tent." It was not until enough people had agreed to join the new sect that they learned they were joining the Seventh-Day Adventists. To Nina this roundabout technique was offensive. She was then and was to remain all her life a direct person. What was good to do, right to do, or necessary to do deserved to be done openly and directly. This was to be part of her strength in later life, and a real part of her charm. There is something disarming and attractive to all the wary and timid of the world in a person who always makes an unself-conscious progression from a beginning to a logical end.

At the close of the summer, a new church consisting of twenty members had been organized.

Nina returned to medical school in the fall. She was so glad to be back that her pleasure was almost pain. She went about her work soberly and earnestly. She and Stella roomed together, but, as far as I know, Stella never again tried to break through to a closer relationship.

In the second year of medical school Nina found that a new element had entered into her relationship with her professors. Somehow, to them, the fact that she was married made her more acceptable; I suppose because it made her seem "womanly." Instead of being a threatening female who aspired to take the rightful bread from the mouth of some male doctor, she was regarded as a dilettante who was playing a game that would end, of course, back in the kitchen and the nursery.

One of the professors made an attempt to establish a more intimate relationship, but he was routed by her innocence. He proposed that he and the "little grass widow" have some fun together. Nina, having no idea what type of "fun" he had in mind, thanked him warmly for thinking of her. She had much too much work to keep up with, she said, to even think of pleasure. But she would enjoy his wonderful lectures even more, now that she knew he was so kind.

The poor professor fled.

Near the end of the school year, when Nina was ex-

periencing an almost physical revulsion at the idea of repeating last year's summer, she was offered an assignment
to work at the medical dispensary back of the stockyards.
The assignment came from the professor in charge of summer work, who had offered the job to every male student
in the second-year class. None of them would take it because the doctor hired to run the dispensary was a woman,
a graduate of the Women's Medical College of Pennsylvania. Nina's living expenses would be paid. The experience in prenatal care she would gain would be of value to
her. She accepted the assignment with joy even before she
wrote to her husband and the church. Fortunately, they all
agreed.

The two women had many problems that summer. They
were frequently out on the streets together at night. Their
patients were poor, undernourished, heedless; miscarriages
were frequent. But the women walked without disaster
through the streets of one of the worst city slums of that
era.

There is something curious and interesting here. In our
day, not long ago, a noted psychiatrist published his theory
about effective self-defense against criminal assault. He
concluded that the weapon that inspired immediate, atavistic, terrifying fear in any human mind, criminal or otherwise, was not a gun or brawn or brass knuckles or an
automobile or a bomb or even an ordinary knife, but a long,
thin, pointed weapon such as an ice pick. Man's courage
when facing a blunt instrument is dangerously misplaced;
but when he is facing a thin, sharp, delicately pointed
weapon, he knows instinctively that his body can be
pierced and destroyed by the weakest hand. Slim, sharp,
delicate destruction can end life without notice and without noise.

Our two women, sweeping the slum dirt from the sidewalks of Chicago with their long skirts, knew this long ago. They made their way along the gaslit night sidewalks with reasonable confidence, fully armed. The hats of those days were trimmed with flowers, feathers, felt, ribbons, bows, velvets, buckles, veils, rosettes. To carry such creations, hair was massed and padded inside with clusters of false hair called "rats." To hold everything together, the hats were anchored to the hair with long, thin, pointed hatpins, each with a sturdy knob at the pushing end. When a threatening figure emerged from the dark shadows, the women stopped under the nearest gaslight and adjusted their hats, pulling out and pushing in the delicate bright metal shafts. Danger faded away into the night.

At the end of a great summer, Nina decided to transfer to the Women's Medical College of Pennsylvania. Her association with the doctor in charge of the dispensary had convinced her that there were more opportunities for women to get firsthand experience in the practice of medicine and surgery there than in a male-oriented medical school. She applied and was accepted; then she informed her husband and the church. Having safely provided for her immortal soul, and having safely located her where she would not be lost, both the church and the Reverend Baierle had, naturally enough, turned to other problems and gratifications. They concurred.

I think we must say goodbye now to Nina the child. She was not yet a woman, but she had developed enough skills of her own to recognize herself as a person. If she was still dependent, she was at least making some decisions and making them firmly, before consultation with authority. Today there is a country-music song that claims there are only three things worth caring about, "old dogs, little children, and watermelon wine." Maybe there's a fourth; maybe it's young adults, beginning persons who will carry on, in the future as in the past, the most fundamental American tradition, a moral force in a jaded, cynical world.

...4

The Women's Medical College of Pennsylvania was founded in 1850. The impetus to establish a medical school for females came from courageous leading doctors in Philadelphia, most of them Quakers, and a handful of brilliant women who had studied with doctor relatives in an apprenticeship relationship and all of whom were denied admittance to existing local schools. They also were denied clinical training in local hospitals. In 1904, the year before Nina transferred to the medical college, Pavilion Hospital was opened by the college. The hospital accepted men, women, and children for medical and surgical treatment. Nina had made a wise move.

Nina was one of three women junior medics who followed Dr. Frederick P. Henry, professor of medicine, down the sun-filled women's ward of Pavilion Hospital. Each of the three students in white coats carried a notebook, a pencil, and a stethoscope. The doctor stopped by a bed, introduced one student to the patient assigned to her, and proceeded on down the ward with the remaining two. Nina was the last to be assigned a patient, a young black girl wasted to a skeleton with fever-bright eyes.

"Martha, this is Dr. Baierle. She will examine you to see if she can find some way to help you."

"All right, Doc. Do you think I'm goin' to git well?"

"You'll be out of here in no time." The doctor's voice was gruff and hearty.

Dr. Henry walked on and left Nina with her first medical case. She looked into Martha's burning, worried eyes and forgot to be self-conscious.

"Do you have pain? Tell me all about how you feel."

"I just feel plumb tuckered out. I'm burnin' up all the time. I thought if only I got enough to eat I'd be all right, but now with lots to eat, I ain't hungry no more."

Nina checked over the chart, checked temperature, blood pressure, pulse, and respiration. She listened to the wheezy, noisy lungs, palpitated the distended abdomen. During every moment of the examination she was searching her mind to remember from her classwork what disease might show the symptoms she was finding. The next morning she repeated the examination and reported to Dr. Henry. With a tremble in her voice, she gave her diagnosis, "galloping consumption."

Dr. Henry broke up. He laughed so loudly that his secretary peered in at the door. His amusement finally subsided enough for him to ask, "And what might that be, speaking in medical terms?"

"Acute miliary tuberculosis." Nina was abashed by the folk term she had used.

"Right you are." Dr. Henry was still smiling. He became grave. "She won't be with you long. I looked in on her early today and she's close to death."

"Dr. Henry! Can't we do something?"

"No. It was too late when she was brought in. She had been too long without food or care. When she is dead you will do an autopsy and confirm your diagnosis, write up your findings, and present them to me with the others you will have during this semester." Noting Nina's troubled face, he added, "Don't worry about it. You'll get used to seeing them die. We can't save them all."

Nina was restless and unhappy after she left the office. She was studying medicine so she could cure her patients, and the very first one was going to die. She went back to the ward and sat down by Martha's bed. In doing so, she was acting exactly as any medical student, even today, acts to help a patient with words when authority, in the guise of the attending physician, has accepted the reality of medical limitations. Anyone who has ever been in a teaching hospital when new medical students start on their first day with their first patients recognizes the intense rejection of experienced opinion that drives the novice back to one patient or another again and again, as though willing the stricken to perform his own miracle.

"You're good to come again," Martha said. "Doc Henry always says I'll git better soon and I don't believe any more. You never say that to me."

"No, Martha, I can't tell you you'll be better soon. Martha, are you afraid to die?"

"Oh, yes, Doc! I'm terrible afraid. I've been bad. I'll go to the bad place sure as hell."

Nina leaned over and took Martha's thin, hot hand. "Listen, Martha, nobody's really good. We're all bad. Only God is good. He is good and very kind. He's looking at you now and He says, 'Martha, you never had a chance. I'm going to let you go to sleep for a little while and then I'm going to give you a new life.' God doesn't see any of us as we think we are. He sees you, now, as you would have been if you'd had a good home, and love, and education. He knows more about your beautiful, patient soul than you know about yourself."

"I like your God," Martha said.

She died just before dawn the next day. Nina went down to the autopsy room, where she did the hardest thing she would ever have to do as a doctor—her first autopsy on her first patient.

...5

In the summer of 1906, between the third year of medical school and her final year, Nina worked at the Barton Dispensary in South Philadelphia. Both the church and Nina's husband again had agreed that the experience would be too valuable for her career to be put aside for summer church work. Her joy in the work she did that summer in the slums of South Philadelphia was double because of her freedom.

On her return to school in September she found that a financial emergency awaited her. Dr. Clara Marshall, dean of the Women's Medical College, had received a letter from the Illinois Conference of the Seventh-Day Adventist Church stating that no further tuition would be paid for Nina Case Baierle by the church. The withdrawal of support was occasioned by a complaint from Dr. Kellogg that Nina had failed to fulfill an oral agreement with him that she would sell his new magazine *Good Health* every summer between school years. Nina was stunned. She was also angry.

Nina's defense of her right to a medical education paid for by the church was white-hot. A record of her response is in the files at the Women's Medical College. She marshaled her defense in depth the way a lawyer assembles his arguments in a case. She began by denying absolutely that she had made any such agreement. She pointed out that had she made such an agreement, the logical time for Dr. Kellogg to claim her compliance would have been at the beginning of one of the two past summers, not at the end of the last summer she would have between school terms.

She then argued that had she made such an agreement

(which she had not), the payment of her tuition was arranged in consideration of her work for the church before
entering medical school and was therefore in no way dependent on any work she might do later. She pointed out
that she had brought in thousands of times more money
than her modest tuition cost by dramatically increasing the
circulation of *Lifeboat*. She made it clear that the salary and
commissions promised her for her *Lifeboat* work, but never
paid, exceeded her medical school expenses. She ended her
defense with a blazing *"I Protest,"* capitalized and under-
lined.

The church backed down. Her tuition was paid for her
final year. But the breach that was to come later between
Nina and the Adventists had its beginnings here. Where
there is only authority and obedience, trust once severely
damaged does not recover its lost purity and force.

Almost before she could believe it, the years of medical
school were over—the grinding study of books on anatomy,
psychology, chemistry, practice of medicine, pharmacol-
ogy, embryology, pathology, surgery, mental diseases,
sanitation; the supervised operations and ward practice;
the laboratory work; all the facts and techniques that
must be learned before controlled intuition can assist
knowledge in the diagnosis and treatment of disease. She
sometimes felt the thought patterns inside her head were
like hemlock boughs in a storm in the forest, everything
moving and waving and tossing in winds from every direction. It was not until early June of 1907, when final examinations were over but graduation day was still a week
ahead, that the time to think about her own future arrived
the way a windless oppressive day sometimes follows a
summer storm.

She seemed to herself to be a stranger in a foreign land.
The church, her husband, and "saving the world" seemed

far away. Even the language of the church seemed to have lost its early comprehensibility. Just as Elder Allen had feared, she had drifted away from a narrow viewpoint. Indeed, the church was right to fear worldly medical schools. And Elder Allen was wrong in trusting that marriage would save Nina from the fate of the young men who had gone to medical school and who had been lost to the church. I think the church had assumed that the Reverend Charles Baierle was maintaining a supportive relationship with his young wife. But Nina's husband had had no relationship with her at all during the past three years. He was a dropout from his assigned task of keeping Nina from becoming lost.

Nina was afraid. It is difficult to leave old ways behind before new paths are clear, but it happens to us all at one time or another. "We wait for light, but behold obscurity; for brightness, but we walk in darkness."

Nina had received a call from the church (a call seems to have been an authoritative order given with no thought of noncompliance) to go to the Seventh-Day Adventist Sanitarium in Melrose, Massachusetts, for further training in obstetrics and surgery. She didn't want to go. The show hospital of the church, Battle Creek Sanitarium, recently had passed out of Seventh-Day Adventist control. The church authorities, depressed and disheartened by the loss, had tightened up medical procedures in the other, smaller sanitariums to conform more strictly with church dogma; new medical practices, which had crept in almost unnoticed, had been banned. What Nina really wanted to do was to live with her husband, open an office for general practice, and start being a doctor free to use all of the healing techniques she had learned. Hoping for support from Charles, she asked him to come for graduation so that they could discuss her future; in her mind, *their* future.

Graduation exercises were held in the Philadelphia Academy of Music. For Nina it was a solemn occasion. When she took the Hippocratic oath, she knew she was joining an order to which she could subscribe without reservation. She took her state boards a few days later and was licensed to practice medicine and surgery.

Charles Baierle had come. He was enthusiastic about her call to Melrose, Massachusetts.

"But what are you going to do?" Nina asked her husband.

"Why, go on with my work, of course! I'll come up to Melrose occasionally; things will work out somehow later on. I have plans that will let us work together. Get all the experience in sanitarium work you can. Watch everything connected with the running of the place. Who knows! Maybe you'll have a sanitarium of your own to run someday."

"I don't want to run anything." Nina was speaking the truth. "I want to open an office and start in private practice."

"This is a poor time to think of such things," Charles said sternly. "You have a great opportunity before you to become a power in the church. How can you wish to work for the world?"

Nina was still a beginning person, still not quite her own woman. Because she was uncertain and afraid, she accepted authority once again.

"I'll go, all right. I'm only thinking I would like to work in a more personal way with patients than just to order baths and diets under the strict rule of a sanitarium."

Charles professed to be shocked at the implied criticism of church policy. He prayed aloud for her that she might feel gratitude to those in authority over her.

A little friendship, a little warmth, a little personal concern sometimes works wonders, but prayer without loving-kindness does not, I think, work at all.

...6

When Dr. Nina arrived at the Seventh-Day Adventist Sanitarium in Melrose, a surprise awaited her. The Leeland family, with whom Nina had lived in Williamsport, were all working at the sanitarium. Brother Leeland was the business manager. Sister Leeland was the dietitian and housekeeper. Myra Leeland was the head of the nursing staff and director of the nurses' training school. Such coincidences occur, but they never cease to create a sense of wonder. It's a small world. The world of the church in those days was indeed small. In any church with a limited number of paid employees, the organizational structure is apt to be heavy on theologians and light on administrators. Brother Leeland was a trained administrator who had proved himself in managing the church's central printing plant. It is not strange that he should be moved periodically to wherever the need for skills in short supply was most acute.

It seemed strange to Nina to be welcomed in Massachusetts by the Leelands of Pennsylvania. There was a short period of awkward readjustment as a different pattern of relationship between them all was established. Nina was no longer the child, the twig that must be bent in the way she should grow. She was Dr. Nina, a member of the hospital staff, which put her near the head of the pecking order. Outwardly, at least, the Leelands treated her with the respect and deference due to her position, although the time was not far off when Brother Leeland would array himself against her and with her enemies.

A unique and distinctive feature of the Seventh-Day Adventist hospitals in those days were the "sanitarium treatments." Modeled on the Kellogg plan, they included hydrotherapy, electrotherapy, various mechanical devices, revulsive treatment by heat and cold for many ailments, electric treatments with galvanic violet ray and static electricity, massage, and, of course, always diet, upon which great emphasis was placed. The use of medicines was allowed, but only those products produced by nature and, of those, only natural medicines that were not habit-forming. The core of the medical staff was made up of Seventh-Day Adventist doctors, but doctors from outside the church were allowed to admit and treat their patients as in any other hospital. Not very many "worldly" doctors sought the privilege. Most of the hospital patients were nervous, stubborn people who had worn out the tolerance of their families, and whose own doctors had put them in the sanitarium out of weariness and professional exhaustion. Some of the patients brought themselves to the sanitarium after being treated by several doctors without benefit. Nina would discover, after she had been at Melrose several months, that very few obstetrical patients came to the sanitarium.

So it was with interest and excitement that she responded to a letter from the matron of the Florence Crittenden Home in Boston. The home, a haven for unwed pregnant girls, had long wished for a woman doctor to handle the obstetrical work of the institution. The matron asked for an interview with Dr. Nina. Nina arranged to go in to Boston.

The two women liked each other on sight. The matron outlined her idea for a small private maternity clinic solely for the use of the girls who lived at the home. The Florence

Crittenden board had purchased an attached building next to the home. The matron proposed to cut doors through on each floor. She envisioned treatment rooms and an office on the ground floor, a delivery room and three patient rooms on the second floor. Thus they could care for the girls and deliver the babies under one roof, without sending the girls out to public hospitals. She had already sounded out two of the members of the Crittenden board and was sure the board would agree to pay for the remodeling. The problem she had not solved was how to equip the clinic once the work was finished.

As the two women wandered around the unused building, assessing its possibilities, Nina found that she wanted a small maternity clinic more than she'd wanted anything for a long time. She had come to Massachusetts for additional training in obstetrics and she wasn't getting it. The students in the sanitarium nursing school had almost no opportunity for experience in obstetrical nursing. It was a serious drawback for them, since most babies were born at home and nurses with obstetrical training were in constant demand.

Nina suggested that the matron get a firm commitment from the Crittenden board to remodel. Nina would propose to her sanitarium board that the hospital undertake to equip the building and arrange for each student nurse to have a month each year at the maternity clinic as a required course before graduation. When she left to go back to Melrose, both women were full of hope and enthusiasm. They were two of a kind, and achievement often grows out of the meeting of like minds.

A week later the matron called. Her board would remodel. The building would be ready in three months. Nina sent her proposal in writing to Elder Herman Bitterman, the chairman of the sanitarium board, along with a request to be allowed to attend the next board session to explain and defend her plan. Her request was granted.

At the meeting, when the subject was opened for discussion, Brother Leeland was the first to object. "How can we take on something like this when we can't get our own institution out of the red?" The sanitarium was not paying its way and the New England Church Conference had to come up with a subsidy each month to make up the deficit.

Nina was ready for the question.

"This clinic will be of real benefit to our nurses' training school. It also will be a wonderful advertisement for our sanitarium to the world. We will gain friends and prestige in medical circles. And it need not cost us a cent. I believe I can furnish the medical equipment for the clinic if I can have two afternoons free each week for the next three months."

"How?" Brother Leeland was skeptical. "Surely you can't do this out of your salary!"

Nina was somewhat bitter about her salary. She was paid $100 a month, but the money was sent to her husband.

"No, I can't. But I've had some experience in selling. I propose to go to manufacturers and merchants and to the benevolent people of the city of Boston. I'll ask for donations of equipment and money."

"That's a big order for one person. It will be a tough job," commented Elder Bidwell, the sanitarium chaplain. "You'll have to have a hot-water heater, bathtub, shower, a tubular treatment table, beds, linens, towels, sterilizers, dressings, rugs, dressers, basins, and many other things."

"I know. I discussed how to manage it with one of the Boston doctors who has a patient here at the sanitarium and who has had a lot of experience with social work in Boston. He tells me that money for the Crittenden Home is relatively easy to raise right now. The wealthy, prominent families of Boston have made a hobby of the Crittenden idea. Helping unwed mothers instead of punishing them, he says, is the newest thing, almost a society fad. Since the maternity clinic will help the home and also will be a training ground for obstetrical nurses, I think I can get the donations."

Elder Bitterman was impressed. He suggested that Nina be allowed to see what she could do in outfitting the clinic. The rest of the board agreed, and she was dismissed from the meeting.

She decided to start immediately. Indeed, she was a little frightened at the scope of the project. She arranged to go to Boston the next afternoon to make a beginning.

Elder Bitterman also was returning to Boston that day to take a train to Worcester, Massachusetts, where he lived with his wife. He invited Nina to share his carriage. Elder Bitterman was not your run-of-the-mill churchman. He was tall and slim, and he wore his fine-quality clothes with the casual suavity ordinarily reserved to sophisticates. At forty-three, he had already made a meteoric rise in the church hierarchy. A convert only seven years ago, he now not only was the chairman of the Melrose sanitarium board but also held the more prestigious office of chairman of the New England Church Conference. He was ambitious. He was charming. He was interested in Nina. He found her amusing and different.

As they rode into Boston, Nina proposed that he head the list of subscribers to the clinic by donating a treatment table, six chairs, and a shower. All of these items were stored unused in the basement of the sanitarium. He decided he had a right, as president of the board, to make such a donation. She immediately put his name and donation down at the top of her subscription list.

During the next three months while Nina was collecting

donations, Elder Bitterman came to the sanitarium with
unusual frequency. He always stopped in Nina's office to
hear about her progress. Sometimes Elder Bidwell accompanied him, but usually he came alone and stayed long,
comfortably chatting. Nina felt she had made a friend—
and a most attractive friend. At the end of three months the
clinic was fully equipped down to a brass sign over the
door. The clinic opened and for the next year Nina, her
nurses in tow, moved back and forth from Melrose to Boston, a busy young woman with interesting work to do. She
delivered fifty-seven babies in the first six months alone,
fifty-seven new lives unwanted by the young mothers who
had conceived them. It was then she realized, she told her
children later, that if she were ever allowed to have children, *she* would want them very much.

The clinic and the sanitarium patients were not her only
preoccupation. Dr. William James, founder of the department of psychology at Harvard and a brother to Henry
James, brought a patient to the sanitarium, a very special
patient, one of the earliest multipersonality cases in psychiatric history. Nina was fascinated with the patient. Dr.
James, whose *Principles of Psychology* had been published in
1890, made her a gift of all his books. He was pleased to
discuss his general ideas with this bright young woman, as
well as to share his views with her about his multipersonality patient.

Mother never said what the other Seventh-Day Adventist doctors and nurses thought about such a patient. *The
Three Faces of Eve* and *Sybil* had not yet made it easy to
believe that more than one personality could inhabit a single body. I would not be surprised if the general opinion
at the sanitarium were that the patient was possessed by
devils. I wonder how many prayers were said, when Dr.
James wasn't there, asking that the demons leave her body

and cast themselves into the nearest running water.

Nina was having a problem about money. The problem was that she had none. She had remonstrated with Brother Leeland about sending every cent of her salary to her husband. Brother Leeland was adamant. Of course her salary should go to her husband. Brother Baierle could then, in his wisdom, decide how much was suitable to return to his wife. The hospital furnished her board, room, laundry, transportation, and uniforms. But the trips back and forth to Boston made it necessary for her to have respectable clothing, and her shoes and gloves and dresses were wearing out.

She started writing stories for a New York newspaper. In those days, many newspapers ran continued stories in their Sunday editions. Inspired by Dr. James's patient, every week she wrote one story, a three- to four-thousand-word episode, called *The Girl with a Hundred Personalities*. She enjoyed the writing, and the paper sent her $10 a week. With Brother Leeland nearby, she said nothing to anyone about her writing project, and kept the current episode on which she was working locked away in her room. She never forgot that he had forced her to burn her first stories.

She also was trying her hand at writing poetry, love poems about loneliness and loss and empty arms. Indeed, Nina was no longer a child. At twenty-four she was about to become a woman at last, even though a naive and inexperienced one, but only after such a grotesque series of events that to become her own person was the only alternative to being nothing at all.

...7

In October, Nina received a summons to appear at the regular monthly meeting of the sanitarium board. When they were all assembled, Brother Leeland opened the discussion. He was never slow to give credit to anyone who had done a good piece of work for a cause that, in his eyes, was worthy.

"I have a suggestion to make. Dr. Nina has done a wonderful job with the maternity clinic. If she can do that, why not let her raise money to lift the burden of debt the sanitarium itself is struggling under?"

"What do you think of that, Dr. Nina? Any ideas?" asked Elder Bitterman.

This was heady stuff for the young woman. Elders of the church, very important persons, deferring to her, asking her opinion. She had to come up with a suggestion, and she did. She proposed that they write to all the Seventh-Day Adventist churches in the New England Conference. Each should arrange a Sunday-night meeting in its locality according to a schedule Brother Leeland would draw up.

"Have them hold the meeting in a public hall, not in the church, and invite the public to come. There should be three speakers at each meeting—Elder Bidwell on 'The Sanitarium Idea,' Elder Bitterman on 'The Clinic Work of the Sanitarium,' and the woman doctor, me, to promote rescue work in the Boston area modeled on the Chicago pattern. A silver offering would be collected to further the work of the Sanitarium Idea."

Her suggestion was received with enthusiasm. After several changes and additions, a motion to proceed was passed by the board. Brother Leeland was instructed to draw up a schedule and send out the letters.

Herman Bitterman spent more and more time at the sanitarium. There is no doubt that he imagined himself to be in love. Charming, ambitious, forty-three-year-old married men often mistake infatuation for something more important than it is. He and Nina were temperamentally suited to each other, and he felt himself to be attractive to her. When his religious beliefs came into conflict with his growing desire to be near her, he could assure himself that nothing had happened and nothing would happen to bring him to actual sin. I doubt if he thought deeply enough about his feelings to realize that a slow drift into an aimless emotional attachment can do great damage even to a mature person. Elder Bitterman's preoccupation with Nina was becoming dangerously close to an actual obsession.

Nina, busy in all directions at once, was not obsessed with him, but she was gratified by his interest in her projects. She really liked the man. One afternoon she arrived back from the Boston clinic to find him waiting in her office, a page of her short poems in his hand. He had been rummaging through the papers on her desk. Nina was terrified for a moment that she had left the latest episode of her newspaper stories where it could be found. She felt great relief that it was poetry. He rose at once.

"I was waiting for you and just happened to look at this writing. I hope you don't mind."

"I'm afraid you've been wasting your time. My writing isn't inspired, you know. It's my way of relaxing."

"This one, 'At the Bird Theatre, Daybreak,' is beautiful. It sounds like a love poem. What does it really mean?"

"Oh, that's something you must see and hear. One night last spring I couldn't sleep so I took a walk around the lake."

"What! Five miles around the lake in the night, alone?" he asked incredulously.

"It wasn't very dark, the moon was full, and I didn't go all the way around. I only got as far as a round hill two miles away, toward Stoneham. I sat down to rest on a log and to watch the first light of dawn. One bird chirped, then another whistled, and almost at once the hill was calling and twittering as though all the leaves of the trees had come alive. There were hundreds of birds. It was the loveliest sound I've ever heard. Later I made up a party—Miss Myra, two other nurses, and several patients. They went with me to hear it. Next year I hope we can take every patient who can walk."

"You like to write, don't you?" he asked. "I would love to read other things you've written. It's a gift. You shouldn't hide it."

The schedule of fund-raising events at every Seventh-Day Adventist church in the New England Conference was soon drawn up, and the three speakers—the chaplain, Elder Bitterman, and Nina—set out for the first of their weekend meetings designed to erase the sanitarium deficit. Each weekend during February and March they were in a different part of New England. Funds began to come in not only from the silver offering but also from larger contributions sent by people who became interested in the Sanitarium Idea. More patients came to the sanitarium.

It was a heady time for Nina. She was generally admired, but it was the increasing admiration of Elder Bitterman that brought a glow to her heart. They were seldom alone together, but when they were, the elder always asked for more of her original work to read in solitude. I suppose that in his state of infatuation, to have something uniquely hers with him during the weekdays of their separation was gratifying. Give me your rose and your glove. Nina didn't think it wise to give him any more of her poetry. She planned to write a series of short articles on religious subjects that would be suitable to dole out to him, but after the first article, which he professed to find enthralling, the demands on her time by the sanitarium, her Boston clinic, and the weekend tours made it impossible to continue turning out new material. When he kept begging for more, she started giving him copies of excerpts from *The Girl with a Hundred Personalities*. She chose mild and general parts of episodes that would not disturb him. She was sure he never read the part of the Sunday paper where continued stories were printed, so she never told him the excerpts had been published.

No human relationship stands still. The status quo between one person and another is impermanent, always shifting toward deeper involvement or toward the blank alienation of indifference. The most delicate and intelligent maneuverings to keep a relationship static fail. Whatever Elder Bitterman had in mind to do with his increasing obsession with the little doctor, chance took the decision out of his hands. The three speakers were returning from their last weekend fund-raising meeting. They arrived by train in Boston early one evening in late March.

At North Station a Western Union messenger boy found them and delivered a telegram to Elder Bidwell. Remember the days of Western Union messengers? They could find anyone anywhere—in stations, trains, hotel lobbies, movie houses. An ingenious bunch of boys who always, with pride, got their man. Elder Bidwell was needed in Lancaster for a funeral. He took the next train out for Lancaster. Nina and Herman Bitterman took the local together for Melrose.

At Melrose they set out to walk the mile and a half to the sanitarium. It was a beautiful night, cold and still, the moon white over the bright, white snow. The road wound through dark-shadowed copses and over little icy, rushing streams. The snow crunched and squeaked under their boots. When the sanitarium came into view they climbed a bypath that would take them to a side door. At the top of the rise, laughing and breathless, they stopped to rest.

"Makes one think of Christmas, doesn't it?" Nina asked.

"It makes me think you're beautiful!" exclaimed Elder Bitterman. He gathered her to him and with gentleness and passion he kissed her. Nina kissed back.

This is not a startling pornographic scene. These two people, booted and heavy-coated, begloved and bescarved and both with hats, had no human contact except for their cold faces and warm lips. For any other two persons, such a scene would not be worth recording. What's a kiss? A pleasant, warming moment for two people who like each other.

But for those two it was shattering. Elder Bitterman's desire was fed at the exact moment when his confidence in being able to remain free from sin was destroyed. Nina learned for the first time that to sexual invitation there can be a chemical response that has a force of its own, ungoverned by moral precepts. Dr. Nina and Herman Bitterman, aghast, stared at each other in the light of the cold moon. Nina turned away, went into the sanitarium, and on to her room.

Elder Bitterman left early the next morning and was seen no more that week at the sanitarium. Elder Bidwell returned on Friday night. It occurred to Nina that a chaplain was one to whom one could go when doubt and confusion depressed body and soul. She decided to confide in Elder Bidwell.

That was a mistake. We all have made the mistake, one time or another, of speaking when silence would have allowed events to straighten themselves out; of confessing to what is better kept hidden from confessors who may act with a dearth of wisdom or an excess of zeal. But how could Nina have known? She was inexperienced in romantic misery and had never transferred an emotional problem to the care of another. With almost incredible naiveté, she told him simply and frankly everything that had happened.

He was reassuring: "My dear, I believe you. I'm sure you had no evil thought. We have made a mistake in making you so prominent and letting you take a man's place. Women in the church should be seen and not heard. It's our fault as much as yours, because I believe you are innocent and unawakened. We will pray that nothing more will come of this."

I can only surmise, in the knowledge of events that occurred rapidly after their conference, that Elder Bidwell, in spite of his prayers, made it inevitable that a great deal would come of this. He must have confronted Herman Bitterman; there is no other rational explanation for what Elder Bitterman did next. Perhaps Elder Bidwell warned him of what would happen if any more nonsense took place —there would be a woe unto Elder Bitterman. In any event, Herman Bitterman asked for a church trial. He acted exactly as many charming, forty-odd-year-old husbands have done when their careers and their domestic tranquillity were threatened; in panic, he decided that his best defense was to attack.

Or perhaps the reason for what happened next is not so simple. Elder Bitterman's decision to ask for a church trial on the charge that Dr. Nina had bewitched him could have been prompted by someone in the church hierarchy whom he had consulted and who was intent on bringing about Elder Bitterman's downfall. The politics among church officials, as among university faculties, can be as sly and convoluted as the politics among contenders for power in the larger national arena.

Or perhaps the ghost of some old New England witch hunter, drifting around in the barren, colorless air of a more rational era, recognized a kindred spirit and urged him into folly. For whatever reason, Elder Bitterman decided to attack. It was a mistake that was to take him all the way to Asia and to make Nina her own person at last.

...8

For the entire week after she talked to Elder Bidwell, Nina went about her work mechanically, in a miasma of despondency and unrest. She was lonely. She also was reassessing her life and her feelings, and assessing what she could rightfully and modestly expect from the future. Nothing was reassuring. She recognized that something was the matter with the life she was leading. Her patients who liked her and responded to her professional care were not her friends; with cure they disappeared. She could not give the benefit of knowledge she had gained in medical school to those patients who were not responding to the strict sanitarium regimen because she was prohibited from applying worldly remedies. Her clinic in Boston was going well. But she had no one to laugh with or have fun with or talk to. And look what happened, she thought ruefully, when I did have someone. She felt herself to be tied up by the church, to be, at age twenty-four, married to the church.

But she was also married to a man. Perhaps there was hope there. She and her husband had had a friendly and courteous relationship; perhaps their relationship could be

broadened and deepened and made a bulwark against loneliness and futility. If both were willing to try, couldn't
their marriage, already sanctioned by the church, be meaningful and rewarding for them both? They could live together. They could have children. If they were never to be
in love with each other, they could learn to love in a different way as they shared the joys and responsibilities of par-
enthood.

In the olden days, in the Bible, she thought, when a man
died his brother or kinsman took up his duties as a husband,
and if children came from the new union, the kinsman
raised the children for his brother in his brother's name.
Few of those bereft women could have been in love with
their brothers-in-law. But the law provided for their right
to have children so that life could go on. Look at the account of Ruth and Boaz. And, she thought, if she had some
human warmth, some human contact with the husband
who was joined with her forever, she would be safe from
the wickedness that lies deep in every human heart, even
in her own.

She decided to ask her husband to come to Melrose. But
on Monday, as she started her morning hospital rounds, she
came face to face with him. What a wonderful coincidence
that Charles should come just when she wanted to talk with
him! Then Nina noticed that he was pale, stern, and tight-
lipped. They arranged to meet at noon after her office
hours.

"How does it happen that you came today?" she asked
when they met outside the nurses' home. Charles had been
grimly pacing the snowy walks.

"I was sent for by the Conference Committee." Nina
looked at him with pleasant inquiry. How her husband's
work in Pennsylvania could be involved with the New
England Church Conference was unclear to her. "You

know very well why I have come," he added with anger. "I've come to attend your trial."

"My trial?" Nina was puzzled. "My trial!" She was alarmed. "What could you mean? I've heard nothing about a trial!"

"Well, you'll soon hear more. The committee meets to-night, and Dr. Alice Hunter came up with me on the train from Washington to take over your work for you while the board's in session."

Nina sank down on a nearby bench. "I don't understand. What have I done? Nothing has happened. My work is going along fine, my patients are getting well, the clinic is doing wonderful work. What can it be?"

Brother Baierle took a letter from his pocket and handed it to her. Dr. Nina kept a copy of it among her notes.

March 10

Brother Charles V. Baierle
Philadelphia, Penna.

Dear Brother Baierle:

I hesitate to write you this letter. A condition of affairs developing out of your wife's actions has created a situation here in the Sanitarium that makes it necessary for the sake of the cause to take action.

The Conference Committee meets Monday evening at 8:00 o'clock in Faneuil Hall, Boston. Your presence is desired. Come as much in advance as you can.

Dr. Alice Hunter has been summoned from Washington, D.C., to take over Dr. Baierle's work while the investigation is going on. She will arrive March 19.

Elder Danforth and Elder Striker of the General National Conference Committee in Washington, D.C., will also attend to advise and counsel.

We want you to know, Brother Baierle, that none of us

hold you to blame for this situation. Dr. Baierle has done some very fine work; she is very talented and has helped to make our work prominent and noticed throughout the New England Conference.

We have learned that she has been writing a series of stories for a New York newspaper that are the most irreligious, heretical writings imaginable, full of earthly passion and wickedness. Judging her from the standpoint of these writings, we can now see what we took for innocent enthusiasm is really an evil influence. We dare not subject our nurses and workers to it.

Elder Bitterman, President of our Conference, has confessed to his wife and to us that he has been spending two-thirds of his time at the Sanitarium, neglecting his work, because he has been bewitched by Dr. Baierle. She has written him the same kind of romantic revelations of her inmost self that has appeared in the stories she writes for the newspaper. This has threatened to undermine his home, his position, and his spiritual life. After much fasting and prayer, he and his wife decided to ask the Conference Committee to help clear it up.

He is putting his life in our hands. While not committing any outward sin, he feels he has betrayed his position, his family, and his God by his unholy infatuation. He has turned over to us the material she has written to him, which will be presented at the meeting.

May God work things out in the right way to save the Sanitarium and the Church from being discredited in any way.

> Sincerely,
> ELDER G. A. BIDWELL

Nina sat on the cold garden bench trying to understand what this monstrous turn of events could mean. She thought of the people she had known who had been cast out

of the church for unsound doctrine, worldliness, or misconduct; she remembered how helpless they had seemed,
and how lost. But sometimes one can be hit too hard to be
helpless and lost; sheer outrage can bring strength. She
turned her thoughts from what the church might or might
not do and, numb with misery, tried to understand Elder
Bitterman. Throughout the rest of her life she was to speak
of him as a moral monster. Long, long afterward she was
to comment bitterly that even Eve had not been accused of
witchcraft.

For Nina, shivering with shock on a cold day, the immediate problem was to remain intact in the face of betrayal,
to decide in a nightmare situation what logical, everyday
steps she should take to prepare for a trial that no one had
had the ordinary humanity to discuss with her in advance.

"It's a wicked lie! What is true in this letter has been
twisted into a wicked lie. You will have to hear about it
from me from first to last. But," she added, as two nurses
came down the frozen walk, "not here. There's a bench
past that big rock near the lake. Go there and wait for me."

Without waiting to see if he would comply with her
abrupt instructions, she turned away, walked back to the
sanitarium, and up to her room. When she returned with
the briefcase that had the clipped-out newspaper stories she
had written, Charles was pacing a snowy walk at lakeside.

It is easy to feel sorry for Charles. He had married a
whiz-kid protégée of the church. He had had every reason
at the time to expect that her brilliance and energy would
carry her to the top of the church structure and he with
her. It would be hard to judge which one of the two was
the more apprehensive and appalled by the strange turn
events had taken. They sat down on a bench, the open
briefcase between them. Nina handed him, one after another, the episodes of *The Girl with a Hundred Personalities*.

He read slowly, gasping now and then with surprise or harumphing with disapproval. When he had read the entire series, she segregated the episodes she had given to Elder Bitterman.

"Read these again," she said. "If Elder Bitterman claims that I wrote any of these for him, you will recognize them as part of an impersonal series."

"I can't understand how you could write such wickedness," the Reverend Charles Baierle said bitterly.

"I had to have money, I just had to have some. I can't apologize for this. I had to buy hairpins, and toothpaste, and equipment to deal with menstruation, and dresses and shoes to wear in public. I have many duties and these stories were the easiest way to make money in the time I had left over. My stories aren't wickedness; they're only imaginative. Forget about them. Our problem is the charge by Elder Bitterman that I have bewitched him. This is a lie. I will never forgive him for this."

As far as I know, even to the day of her death, she never did.

"I'm hungry, and you look ill," Brother Charles said. "I'll go up and bring us down some lunch. We'll talk this over." His voice was kind.

The hint of kindness was almost too much for logic and strength. Fortunately, he had already left, so she could gather herself together by herself. She had time to pray. All she could pray for was that God would help her husband to believe what was true so that she would not be entirely alone in her own defense.

Seldom has a prayer been so swiftly answered. When Brother Baierle returned to the cold bench with cold sandwiches and cold milk, he said, "I believe you. I'll stand by you in this thing as much as I can without endangering my position in the church. I'm sure that the others will see this in the right light. We'll go to Boston today. I'll attend the meeting tonight, which will be only an organizational session for your trial. That will start tomorrow. We'll stay in Boston until this is over."

...9

The Reverend Charles and Dr. Nina arrived early at the meeting room for the trial. Mother later would tell her children that she had insisted she and Charles be the first to arrive because she preferred to watch the elders assemble rather than make a late entrance into a hostile group of old men. We agreed with her that this was a canny maneuver. According to Mother's notes, Elder Bidwell was the next to arrive, followed almost immediately by the elders from Washington, Striker and Danforth. They spoke to Nina and asked Charles to join them at the far end of the room. There they huddled in a circle, talking earnestly together in low tones.

Next came Elders Eldress, Atlee, and Buchanan, then Brother Leeland, followed by Elders Rustman, Jones, Kerby, and Banks. Last, Elder Bitterman came with his wife and with white-haired Elder Carson. The chairs had already been arranged in the center of the room in a semi-circle. Nina and Charles were seated on the left end and Herman and his wife on the right end. The two couples faced each other directly.

Elder Danforth, from Washington, led in a long solemn prayer. Elder Bidwell stated the case against Nina. Elder Striker, obviously the Important Person from Washington, called upon Elder Bitterman to testify. Herman began. Whenever he hesitated in outlining the methods used by

Nina to bewitch him, his wife would interrupt: "Now tell how she tempted you. Tell how you had to fight her off!" Nina's notes of the trial contain a lot of talking by Sister Bitterman. No wonder Herman spent two-thirds of his time at the sanitarium. His testimony took up the long morning past the usual noon dinner hour. The trial was adjourned until the following day.

On the second day of the trial the newspaper stories were presented. Herman Bitterman presented them. He had read only two episodes when he was interrupted by Elder Striker.

"May I ask Elder Bitterman what possible relationship these stories have to the subject under discussion? Is the doctor on trial for writing stories for a newspaper, or for misconduct with you?"

A startled ripple went around the semicircle. Brother Leeland, who honestly believed imaginative writing was inspired by the Devil himself, turned red with holy wrath when what he accounted to be a corruptive activity was so lightly put aside.

Sister Bitterman said, "Herman is only trying to show what an evil mind this woman has."

Elder Danforth backed up his colleague from Washington. "I think Elder Striker has a point. I move that we dispense with further reading of these articles. Most of us have read the whole series. Both Elder Striker and I receive the Sunday newspaper in Washington from New York. We have both found these stories to be amusing and, what's more important, clinically interesting. We were both students of Dr. William James at Harvard, and I, for one, have wondered who the author was."

"I might add," Elder Striker said, "that we stopped in New York on the way here and talked to the editor of the newspaper."

"What did he say?" asked Elder Bidwell.

"He refused to divulge the name of the author. We are not even sure that Dr. Baierle is the writer of these stories. They seem much too clinically accurate for so young a woman to write. Do you have any positive proof, Elder Bitterman, that she wrote these articles?"

"Yes, I have. When you hear the letters she wrote to me you will see that they're the same kind of thing." Elder Bitterman was shaken. The trial had taken an unexpected turn. He had not expected the men from Washington to have any information at all. Many people, before and since, have underrated intelligent, knowledgeable people from Washington.

"One question, Elder Bitterman, before you begin," said Elder Striker. "Were these letters mailed to you?"

"No. She gave them to me on different occasions when I was in her office."

"Very well. Proceed." Elder Striker turned his head and smiled at Dr. Nina, a warm, friendly smile. She had sat quietly throughout the trial, her face pale even to the lips with strain and suppressed indignation. With that smile, hope ruffled in her heart the way a dove, warm and plump and rosy, settles into her nest.

Elder Bitterman droned on, reading what he now recognized was known to be published, impersonal material. He wiped his forehead often with a fine linen handkerchief.

"Now, Dr. Baierle, we will hear your side. What have you to say?" Elder Bidwell's voice was pontifical.

Dr. Nina stood. Soberly she looked at Elder Bidwell and then at each of the elders in turn. The silence was prolonged into embarrassment for everyone but Nina. She was momentarily unaware of what she was doing as a physical body, because into her mind, full-blown, had come her father's voice as he backed Elder Bates out of the door, past the chip pile, and through the garden gate, all those years ago. She had not known, then, what the words he used meant. She was never to remember them again. But at that moment she heard his voice complete. Looking around at the solemn faces of the elders, she could think only of how profoundly shocked they would be if she said what her father had said. Red came back into her lips, her cheeks flushed, her eyes sparkled, and she laughed.

Mother had an amazing laugh. There was no titter and no shrillness. The only analogy that comes close to describing her laugh is the sound of a finely made, artfully arranged Japanese wind chime blown suddenly by a strong gust of wind that makes the glass prisms peal and ring and go beyond a tinkle into a beautiful, irresistible sound of joy.

The elders were shocked. Before they could shake themselves out of their surprise, Nina sobered.

"No, I have nothing to say to you, now or ever. I thought that you, Elder Bidwell, and you, Brother Leeland, and you, Elder Bitterman, were holy men of God. I now think you are disgusting!" She swept to the door, retrieving her coat and gloves as she went, and left the scene.

...10

Back in her room at Melrose, Dr. Nina furiously packed her belongings. She told her children later that she felt, that night, like the ice maiden of the fairy tales, frozen with rage. She acted without caution, without fears, without the nagging regret for the past that ultimately dissipates red-hot anger. Nothing could stop her advent into a new life —not her sanitarium patients, her clinic, her ties with the past years of her life. She felt as inexorable as a glacier.

She had realized, on the train from Boston, that she had never joined the church. Baptism was a basic requirement for membership in the sect, and she had refused baptism when she was nine years old. She had no honest obligation to go farther along the road that led away from the life she needed.

The next morning Charles went to the staff dining room for breakfast. When Nina didn't appear, he went to her room and knocked at the door. She was dressed. She was finishing her packing.

"What goes on here?" Charles asked, surveying the suitcases and packing boxes.

"I'm leaving here with you today."

"Nina, you can't do that! I would have told you last night, but when I looked in after I returned from Boston, you were sleeping. Your trouble is over. The committee has dismissed all charges. Of course," he added, "no one is pleased about your writing. That will have to stop." Nina continued with her packing, saying nothing. "Aren't you glad? Don't you want to hear about it?"

"Yes, I'm glad that at last I am free of their domination. I'll never work another day for any of them, now or ever."

"But wait until you hear what happened after you left!"

The details of the conclusion of Dr. Nina's trial are third-hand, from Charles to Mother to me. He reported that the entire committee had sat in amazed silence after Dr. Nina closed the door behind her. Elder Striker was the first to speak.

"In this whole trial, there has been nothing solid but the confessed infatuation of Elder Bitterman, a man almost old enough to be Dr. Nina's father. There is not a word in these so-called letters that was not already in the newspapers. On my part, it seems to me to be inconceivable that any of these were written to him at all. What do you say, Brother

Baierle? You're more involved in this than any of the rest of us."

The Reverend Charles proceeded to give them Nina's account to him. He was encouraged to support his wife by the nods and echoes of agreement of those church dignitaries more important than he.

Elder Bidwell repented of his role. "I feel as though scales had dropped from my eyes. The worst I can see is that Dr. Nina let her imagination run wild. I'm sorry I had such a big part in this miserable business. I move and cast my vote for not guilty."

The motion was seconded and the vote was unanimous.

"Brother Baierle, please convey this decision to your wife. Elder Bitterman's case will be taken up later by the Conference Committee." Elder Bidwell, Charles reported, carefully refrained from looking at the Bittermans, who had risen after the vote and were on their way to the door.

"When Elder Bidwell and I had put the elders from Washington on the train," Charles said, "we had time to talk on the local coming back to Melrose. Elder Bitterman will never be in charge here again. He's to be sent to Asia as a missionary."

"I'm sorry for his wife. She won't like that at all." Nina paused to be sad as she viewed the wreckage of their association. "But I can't care about any of them. Don't you want me to come with you?" A young, wistful, please-say-yes-if-you-can note came into her voice.

"No." Brother Baierle was unmoved. "You'd better remain here for another year. I need the money; I'm not ready to have you come. The private sanitarium building I'm getting ready for you in Mt. Pocono, Pennsylvania, won't be ready until next spring. Twelve hundred dollars more will help."

So that's what he was doing with her salary. It was a

curious aberration in both of Mother's husbands—both were to build her a hospital she didn't want. She wanted to be a doctor, not an administrator. She had a total aversion to record keeping. She would write prescriptions, fill out birth certificates and other necessary medical forms, and that was as far as she would go. Later, when she had money, she wouldn't even fill out check stubs. When her canceled checks came from the bank, she gave the checks and her checkbook to her accountant. Record keeping was his business, not hers. In the later years of her life she was to drive the Internal Revenue Service mad with frustration. The IRS sent so many young men up from Washington to try to mend her ways that they all became, to Dr. Nina, her friends. She always invited them to stay to dinner. Her conscience was clear, her records were nonexistent, and her cooking was superb. She enjoyed the IRS and never could understand why, after a particularly nice young man had gone through her desk, her cashbox, her medical records, and her accountant, Herb Crane, she would get long, reproving letters from the Internal Revenue Service in Washington. Sometimes she didn't even open the letters.

But whether she did or did not want to run a hospital was not the immediate problem.

"I'm sorry to disappoint you, Charles, but I'm leaving here today, with or without you. I am resolved. I'm a qualified doctor licensed to practice not just here but also in Pennsylvania. On the train we can talk over plans for me to make money."

"Don't be hasty, Nina." It was the Reverend Charles whose voice was pleading now. "I'll send Elder Bidwell to talk to you."

"Don't you dare! Don't you send any of them. I'll talk to no one. Go collect what they owe me and order a cab for the train."

Brother Baierle went. We have a woman here, with a vengeance. No brave child, no conforming adolescent, no beginning adult. A real person.

When they were on the train she told him bluntly of her plan to have a family. Brother Baierle rebelled.

"See here, Nina! You can't be in earnest. What would we do with a family? How could you work, burdened with a baby? Please don't spoil everything now. I've spent a lot of time and money fixing up a place for you to work. It would all be ruined if you had a baby. I can't understand what's come over you. The Lord is coming soon. His people, especially the leaders, should be above things of the flesh. We should not have children in these last days."

Nina laughed.

"That's really funny. There isn't time for us to have a home and a family because the Lord is coming soon. But we have plenty of time to build and run a sanitarium! I think you don't have the slightest idea how much time and work it will take to start making money with a private hospital. Even the church-supported hospitals operate at a deficit. I'm willing to try, but in return I'm going to have a family. If not yours, then someone else's."

Brother Baierle shook his head in bafflement. "How you've changed in the last few years! You used to put the Lord's work first; now you sound sacrilegious. What *is* the matter with you?"

For the next half hour he stared out the train window. When he turned back he was, to Nina's surprise, quiet and helpful. They decided she should open an office for private practice in Scranton, Pennsylvania, to help finish the sanitarium. Brother Charles offered to visit the church in Scranton to find her a room with one of the church members. She refused. She would find an office with room enough for sleeping quarters. She would accept the members of the church as patients, but that would be the limit of her association with them.

"You'll feel differently after a while. Don't let this experience make you bitter or separate you from God," he cautioned solemnly.

"I have no intention of being separated from God. I intend to be what God meant me to be: a doctor, a wife, and a mother. I'll keep my part of our bargain; as soon as the sanitarium is finished, I'll expect you to keep yours."

She meant it; a contract is a contract. Each performs his part of the deal. But how did she make sure that he would perform his? I feel it is somewhat unseemly for a daughter to be curious about her mother's sex life. But how can one help wondering? Can a man be ordered into one's bed? Nature has a simple way of countermanding such an order. How did she manage? Imagine a virgin ordering into her bed a man whose duty it is to make love to her, even though he finds her unattractive, and to do so for the express purpose of impregnating her, although he dislikes children and wants none of his own. Imagine. I'd rather walk, singing hymns, by a panther.

PART
FIVE

---

*"And the the darkness shall turn to dawning,
and the dawning to noonday bright."*

...1

Little Dr. Nina was happy. As she traveled the streets of Scranton in her rented horse and buggy, she sang softly to herself. Her practice, so slow at first that she often went to bed hungry, had increased until now she was able to pay for her office, with a cot in a small back room; to buy enough food; and to send a regular hundred dollars a month to Charles for the sanitarium building. The building itself had been completed three months ago; the delay in opening was only a wait for the last of the equipment to arrive. But Nina had claimed Charles's half of the bargain the day the builders had finished building. He had come, she was no longer a virgin, she was pregnant. Good for Charles! She was so happy, the whole world looked to her like a Christmas tree with lights—a thing she had seen only through other people's windows. In the Seventh-Day Adventist Church in those days, Christmas wasn't celebrated. The teaching was that the day of Jesus' birth was deliberately shrouded in mystery so that worldly celebrations could not distract His people from their primary purpose: to spread the truth about His second coming. She dreamed about the Christmases to come with a tree, green and aromatic, softly glowing on the faces of her children.

She was also eating forbidden fruit; forbidden meat, to be more accurate. One day a week she went to a restaurant to eat, each week a different restaurant, until she had located the cooks in Scranton who, at a reasonable price, prepared food with understanding and care. She no longer chose a vegetable dinner with the added request for as little seasoning as possible; she liked and respected vegetables and always ordered five or six with every dinner, but the big adventure was meat. She ate roast beef, steak, lamb chops, mountain trout, chicken, turkey; sometimes her heartbeat was so rapid at her own daring that she could hardly swallow. She ordered coffee and drank it; she ate dessert without caring if the crust had or had not been made with lard. She still would not order pork, but years later, when we were all feasting on her gourmet cooking and blandly assuming that everyone ate so well, she cooked succulent hams, and a roast pork dish with red cabbage, tart apples, red wine, spices, and chestnuts that could make strong men faint with anticipation before dinner was announced.

One day she passed a nickelodeon. She stopped. She decided she should see a moving picture show—not for herself, she reasoned, but for the sake of her children. They would do everything she had never done, see everything and know everything so that each one would find her own path to Heaven. She herself should know enough about worldly things to guide them away from actual danger. She bought a ticket and went to the door. There she hesitated. She turned back and said to her guardian angel, in her mind, Please wait for me! She laughed; of course guardian angels waited. That was their job. If mortals went into an evil place, the angels folded their wings over their faces and waited outside with infinite patience until they could go on with their guardian work. She gave the ticket to the usher, enjoyed the piano music and the moving picture, and found no wickedness at all.

As her viewpoint on religious observances changed, she began to feel more at home in the world. She was no longer a stranger. Her patients and their families became her friends. Wherever she went she was treated with the natural courtesy the unself-conscious and candid people of the world draw out from others. She had rejected once and for all the church tenet that Heaven was an exclusive place where only one sect could enter, so she could feel kinship with anyone who needed her. The response was beautiful. Her patients trusted her, followed her instructions, and in partnership with Dr. Nina, recovered health. The boys at the livery stable, the waitressess at the restaurants where she ate, the patrolman outside her office on Wyoming Avenue in Scranton watched out for her and worried if she broke her routine. However small it was, however tentative, she had made a place for herself in an increasingly friendly world.

When the last of the equipment was installed, the sanitarium was opened. Dr. Nina had seven patients, although there were private rooms for twelve. Five were obstetrical patients, one had jaundice, and one was "nervous." The nervous patient was over sixty, a pleasant, reasonable woman whose only nervous trait was a recurring disdain for wearing clothes. Her daughter and son-in-law and their children had been getting more and more nervous themselves as Grandma, who lived with them, appeared more and more often at dinner, even when there were guests, clad only in her pale-white, aging, sagging flesh.

The hospital was located somewhat outside the then tiny town of Mt. Pocono, and just on the edge of a privately owned property locally known as the Devil's Hole. The entire tract encompassing the Devil's Hole, more than five hundred acres of forest land, had been bought by a New York banker, enclosed by a chain-link fence, and stocked with Canadian elk. No one now knows why the owner wanted an elk preserve of his own, but there the elks were, hundreds of them, in a compound already becoming inadequate for their numbers. The fence was intended to keep the animals in, not to keep people out, so the gates were never locked. Local people often came on summer Sundays to walk around inside the preserve, feeding indigestible goodies to the elk, which, like goats, seemed willing to eat anything. Until, that is, the sixth spring, when the male elk, fully matured, turned out to be dangerous animals. A local farmer, wandering around the preserve counting fawns born during the early spring, had been attacked and killed by a male elk's flashing hoofs. From then on, anyone coming too near the fence itself was apt to hear the thunder of hoofs as the males rushed to the defense of their small territory.

The routine at the hospital settled down. The wife of a nearby farmer came every day to do the cleaning, and her husband, Phil Utterback, did the mowing and wood-chopping outside in his spare time. Charles installed two church members, Brother and Sister Sinkler, in a log cabin on the property. Brother Sinkler acted as hospital orderly and admittance officer. Sister Sinkler was supposed to do the cooking, but she was a dismal cook. Dr. Nina took over, with Sister Sinkler as her chief assistant and kitchen helper. Charles was seldom home; he appeared only briefly between preaching engagements and Bible study with groups around the state.

Nina would rise early, cook a good breakfast for the staff and the patients, make rounds, borrow Phil's horse and buggy to make house calls on outpatients in the area who had come to her sanitarium office for help. She would cook a big dinner at noon, check her patients, hold outpatient office hours, and fix a supper of soup and homemade bread with homemade applebutter, preserves, and cheese. In the evenings, before her last patient check, she made baby clothes. With all the fresh air and good food, twenty-five-year-old Dr. Nina grew rounder and rosier and happier with every day that dawned. Obstetrical patients came and left with their babies, other medical patients came and went, the nervous woman became such a fixture in the little establishment that even Phil, working outside, would lead her back in to his wife or Sister Sinkler or Dr. Nina when she wandered out, naked as Eve, pleasant and gracious and willing to be led back to the unwanted clothes.

But one night, during the last bed check, Dr. Nina found the woman gone. Her nightgown was on the floor. Everyone else slept, so Dr. Nina went out into the bright-lit full-moon night to retrieve her patient. She searched, but it was not until twenty minutes later, as she quietly neared the elk preserve, that she saw her. There the woman was inside the fence in an open glade, dancing in the moonlight, her white skin gleaming, and around her in a full circle the shining, terrified eyes of dozens of wild, mature elk. Dr. Nina opened the gate latch without a click. Slowly and quietly, keeping on the path to the glade to avoid twig noise, she walked up to her patient, took the woman's hand, and slowly, without a word, led her, still dancing, back up the path. The nearby elk, their opaque eyes flashing as they wheeled to watch, breathed hoarsely in fright. Nina slammed the gate behind her with a bang, knocked the latch down with a loud click, and the spell broke. The elk came thundering to the fence, their towering, muscled chests bowing out the strong unyielding wire. "For thou hast been a strength to the poor, a strength to the needy in his distress, a refuge from the storm, a shadow from the heat, when the blast of the terrible ones is as a storm against the wall."

...2

The first time there was an inkling in Dr. Nina's mind that there were serious difficulties in her marriage was when she happily announced to Charles that she had arranged to have no patients at the hospital from a week before her baby was due until three weeks after the birth. Charles went into a black rage. No kindness and courtesy then; shouting and recrimination and bitterness.

"I told you it was foolish to have a child. You wouldn't listen! You said a baby wouldn't keep you from working and already, before it's even born, it's crippling your work!"

"It's only for a month that I won't be working." Nina was astonished by the bitterness in his face.

"You'll never be able to run a place like this with a baby. We'll be ruined! You'll spoil all my plans because of your stupid idea of having children." Charles was so angry he sputtered and choked.

He was even more angry when he found that she intended to go to Philadelphia for the birth so that Dr. Tenant, of the Department of Obstetrics of the Women's Medical College, could attend her. Nina, having no money of her own except the amount she had put away to pay Dr. Tenant, and knowing that Charles would never agree to pay for a room at Pavilion Hospital, where she longed to be, had arranged with Dr. Tenant and Charles's sister, Caroline, for a home delivery at Caroline's house. Charles washed his hands of the whole problem, packed his valise, and went away.

It's hard to make Charles Baierle seem real because he is

not very real to me. Our ways parted before I was three years old, so there are only flashes of special events involving my natural father that can be called to mind, even with intense concentration. He was a preacher and a church worker full time and an artist in his leisure time. I hold the theory that he would have been a happier and more competent human being if he had been a full-time artist. One small oil that has survived the divorce and the years since then shows real merit. The discipline imposed by work necessary to perfect a talent, even a small one, might have given strength and purpose to what, perhaps unfairly, has always seemed to me to be his rather weak and opportunistic character. Moreover, he often received a "call" to fresco the altar walls of new Seventh-Day Adventist churches, tiny white churches in Pennsylvania, Maryland, and New York. Fresco is a demanding technical artistic medium. I remember well the huge figure of Christ at his second coming, complete with angels in glory, on the altar wall of the little church that was once on Second Street in Strouds-burg, Pennsylvania. The colors were Raphael-like, salmon pink, tender blue, burnished gold; and the shadings in the blowing robes and in the cherubs' wings seemed to me then to be miraculous.

Charles and his older sister, Caroline, had been brought to this country as small children by their Bavarian parents. I have met other Germans from Bavaria and some have struck me as being excessively metaphysical, overly mystical, and too often willing to con others into assuming their practical problems. Charles had chosen to be a preacher, perhaps so that his occupation, involved as it was with theology and supramundane concerns, could put him firmly above onerous daily annoyances. He was an emotional speaker who regularly reduced the congregation to tears. He had a beautiful voice.

It is easy to see, looking back, that this marriage was not made in Heaven. Neither Charles nor Dr. Nina could remotely understand the other. Nina was to learn, slowly and with pain, that no matter how energetically and imaginatively she tried to bring it about, he would never love her. Charles was to learn, with fright and distaste, that she intended they should love each other no matter how long it might take to begin.

The baby, Roberta, was born with great difficulty. Nina was too small to have any baby easily, especially the first one. She also reacted badly to the anesthesia, which had to be discontinued during the hardest part of the birthing. For two days after her little girl was born, Nina hovered between living and dying, semiconscious. Then she began to mend. Her recovery was slow, but at the end of three weeks, after Caroline had notified Brother Sinkler to cancel all patient admittances for another month, Nina packed her satchel, dressed the baby in her prettiest clothes, and took the train from Philadelphia home to Mt. Pocono. She was so exhausted when she arrived that she went immediately to bed. Charles, who had arrived two days before from Bible study in New Jersey, found the baby uninteresting, even in her prettiest clothes.

Charles was upset by the delay in reopening the sanitarium. He stalked about tight-lipped and glowering. He tried to persuade Nina that one more week would be long enough for her to loll about, but the doctor knew more about the state of her recovery than the preacher. He was furious.

"I guess you don't want to help me. You look as strong as ever. Having a baby oughtn't to cripple a woman forever. Indian women had their babies and caught up with the tribe and helped with the work the next day!"

"I read a lot about Indians in California," Nina said.

"They were magnificent! American Indians have a great physical heritage. I've often wished I were part Indian."

Charles, unconvinced and resentful, left the next day to preach on Saturday in Allentown, where he planned to remain until Sunday night.

Sunday was a lovely July day. Brother and Sister Sinkler had gone to visit one of their daughters; Mr. and Mrs. Utterback were at their farm; Nina and Roberta were alone on a summer day gold with sun and flowering wild mustard, a day of olfactory brilliance with red wild phlox mixing the dense, sweet scent of their heavy, multiflowered heads with the dry, clean smell of the golden hay ready for mowing in the big meadow between the hospital and the railroad tracks.

Nina had bathed the baby and was feeding her when she heard a crackling noise. In the olden days in the country, before electricity, outside noises were all more evident and less ominous than now; a farm cat stalking a field mouse through dry grass would crackle through an open window. Nina's mind only noted the noise, but ten minutes later she was aware of a roaring sound, like a big wind blowing around a house corner. She glanced out of the window, thinking a storm must be brewing, but the sun was shining brightly and no branch moved. She put the baby on the chair and went to the back of the sanitarium. As she approached a back window, she was aware of intense heat.

Through the window she could see great billows of black smoke curling over the meadow, and she saw something running down the windows. With horror she realized that what appeared to be water was actually melted glass dripping from the upstairs windows. The entire top story at the back of the sanitarium was on fire. It had been constructed from secondhand lumber salvaged from abandoned houses in the area, and a fire started by sparks from a passing train had swept across the ripe hayfield and had found ready tinder in the dry wood. Nina raced back to the baby and out the front door. She met trainmen from the railroad and neighbors rushing up the road. There was not much anyone could do except put out spot fires catching in the woods surrounding the blazing sanitarium.

So Mother's first hospital burned down. One would surmise that from then on she would have been freed from the onerous burden of being what she had no intention of becoming, an administrator and record keeper. But she would have a second husband whose first act of love would be to build her yet a second hospital. That which she most feared kept coming upon her.

She and Charles and the baby repaired once again to Caroline's house in Philadelphia. Charles was exuberant, all kindness and courtesy. The building and equipment had been fully insured, and he had already received an astonishingly generous offer from the New York elk man to buy the land to enlarge his preserve. Nothing could be finer for Charles than to be free of worry and to have considerably more money than he'd ever had before. The insurance company, with the usual grumping delay and bureaucratic reluctance, paid off in September, two days before the settlement with the New York banker took place. The next week, Charles announced that he had decided to take a trip around the world.

...3

In 1911, this was an astonishing announcement. Nina, now twenty-six, and Caroline, over fifty, were equally astounded. Today, many of us have been around the world, and up and down and catty-corner from far place to far place. Those of us who have traveled less know many people who have seen it all. But in 1911 in the small steamships, the great ocean was truly great and dangerous and the trip seasickening and interminable. Throbbing, churning machinery broke down and help was not easily found in the lonely lanes of the heaving sea. Babies were born and sick passengers died and were gravely dumped into the salt water to feed the fishes, a whole era of each life was given over to the effort to survive the difficult journey. Charles suddenly became a very surprising and foolhardy man to his wife and sister.

It became clear, however, that he didn't mean what he said. He wasn't going "around the world," he was going to Europe and the Holy Land and to Egypt. Charles's mind was imprecise. He planned to write a series of lectures on Palestine and Egypt. Nina was bewildered.

"What are the baby and I supposed to do while you're gone?" Nina knew that a trip of that sort in those days would take at least a year to accomplish.

"With part of the insurance money, I've already arranged for a new house to be built in Delaware Water Gap. I designed it myself. The materials have already been bought and the contractor paid. It will be ready in the spring. You and Caroline can live together until then. I'll leave some money in the bank for your share of expenses. When you move to the new house, you can start working again. If you can't find anyone to take care of Roberta, you can take in two or three patients to make ends meet until I come back." Charles was handy at planning the lives of others to suit himself, but probably no more selfish and autocratic than other men of his era. "I've been terribly upset by this whole thing—the fire, and all my plans destroyed. I need a vacation." He intimated that when he came back, they might start a new life together.

The night before he was to sail, Charles forgot about waiting until he returned. He came into Nina's bedroom. Charles was becoming worldly indeed. Nina put aside the resentment she must have felt for his surliness and his rejection of their child; she was always single-minded when reaching toward a goal. She was still intent on the achievement of love between them. She may even have been heartened that he came on his own decision to her bed. And there is no doubt that Nina was sexy, the quality of passion given to some is not lacking in one sphere while being manifest in all others.

Charles sailed away "around the world," leaving no itinerary. In those days before travel agencies, once the mighty ocean was behind them, travelers crossing Europe disappeared for months as they worked their way with on-the-spot railroad reservations past hostile borders and through the primitive Balkans. Once Charles arrived in the Middle East, any letters he might write would have been mailed from places he had already left. He would be unreachable until his return.

Nina went to Gimbel's bank, where her husband had his account, and presented a check, Charles's bankbook, and his withdrawal card. It was the first time she had ever been in a bank. She was awed. The teller took her documents and went away. When he returned, he was grave.

"I'm sorry. Mr. Baierle withdrew all his balance in this account last week. He opened a savings account, but he left no money in the checking account. The account is closed."

"I don't understand! He said he left money for us. He's gone on a trip to Europe," Nina said earnestly. She was sure if the teller could understand the problem, he would solve it.

"I'm sorry. That's too bad. Maybe you misunderstood;

maybe he left money in some other bank." The teller looked at her intently.

Mother was always sure he thought she was trying to get money that didn't belong to her. She was dreadfully embarrassed. I doubt that he was suspicious. The sight of a beautiful and respectable young woman bewildered by a financial problem must have engaged his sympathies as much as any teller's sympathies can be engaged. Nina left the bank and sat in a nearby coffee shop to absorb her new problem. She had a small reserve of money made up from checks given as gifts by friends and patients for the new baby. There was no point in worrying Caroline with the problem. Caroline adored her younger brother, and besides, she lived on a pittance left to her by their parents; what possible help could Caroline be? Nina would have to find a job. She was forlorn.

The job-placement office of the Women's Medical College was always helpful to the graduates of the institution. Nina consulted with them, and a week later she was appointed resident physician at the Barkman Dispensary in the slums of South Philadelphia. She would receive board, room, care of the baby, and $25 a month.

Caroline was, naturally, indignant.

"Haven't you job enough taking care of your baby? You can't turn Bobby over to the care of strangers for twenty-five dollars a month!" The baby, Roberta, had already been nicknamed Bobby, a name she is still called.

Mother was always sorry she did not feel free to tell Caroline the real reason for the move. All she could do was point out that the experience she would gain in obstetrics, other young women doctors would be glad to pay for. She moved to the dispensary, leaving a disgruntled and disapproving Caroline behind.

Six weeks after Dr. Nina took charge at the Barkman

clinic, she finally had to admit to herself that she was pregnant again. She wasn't sorry; she wanted children, and
pregnancy was a boon to her health. In those days pregnant
women stayed indoors out of sight, but Dr. Nina's patients
were poor, undemanding, and pregnant with her. They
enjoyed having a pregnant doctor.

She worked as long as she could and saved every cent she
earned. Two weeks before her baby was due, Nina took
Bobby and their belongings on the train to Stroudsburg,
where she had decided to open a practice. She had arranged
to live with a Mrs. Mary Kotz, on Ann Street, until the
baby was born and Nina was well enough to move into the
just-completed Delaware Water Gap house. Mrs. Kotz's
niece, Mary McNeal, called Mame, was to be little Dr.
Nina's lifelong friend, a woman of good humor, sturdy
common sense, and strong opinions, all in favor of her
friends and her kin. No fact could ever cause her to question the virtue, the rectitude, and the right to special consideration of anyone in either of those groups. Would that
each of us could have such a friend! Dr. Nina arranged with
the town's oldest and most respected doctor to attend the
birth.

On a warm spring day at the end of May, when labor
began, the doctor was called. He harnessed his horses to his
carriage, and on arrival began immediately to assist in the
birth. Dr. Nina was horrified; he smelled of stables and
leather and he had not stopped to wash his hands. She
suggested, between pains, that he do so. He pooh-poohed
such city nonsense. He had delivered hundreds of babies
without newfangled notions. He cut the cord with unsteril-
ized scissors dug out from the bottom of his black bag, and
left with all seeming to be well. Two days later the baby
began showing signs of an infection around the umbilical
cord. On the third day Dr. Nina, frantic with concern, rose

and dressed and took the baby to Philadelphia. Everything that could be done was done at the Pavilion Hospital, but not much in those preantibiotic days was helpful. The baby died.

Nina borrowed enough money from friends at the Women's Medical College to pay for his funeral and to get her through the first three months of the new office she planned to open in Stroudsburg. The baby was buried on a balmy June day. The sun shone through the trees at Woodlawn Cemetery, making patterns on the bright green grass. Nina sat by the graveside after the little white casket had been lowered into the ground. She thought of her mother's baby; she thought of the baby born to King David and the widow of Uriah, the man whose death David had so cruelly arranged; she thought of all the babies born in the slums of Chicago and Philadelphia, all the babies who had had life for such a brief moment of time, and she wept bitter tears for them all.

...4

Thackeray once said that nature has written a letter of credit upon some men's faces which is honored wherever it is presented. That was in the olden days; nowadays, one has to prove by other documentation who one is in order to get a signed, valid plastic credit card accepted. Who looks at faces any more? But in Stroudsburg, Pennsylvania, in July of 1912, little Dr. Nina got credit for everything she needed. She and her little girl had moved into the newly completed house on a hill above the village of Delaware Water Gap. She had bought a bed, a crib, a stove, pots and pans, and one chair, all on credit. She had found a small office in Stroudsburg, the nearest town on the trolley line, and, with the money she had borrowed, paid the rent for three months. She went to the Stroudsburg National Bank. She was too intent on arranging a loan for office equipment and furniture to be awed by the second bank she had ever entered. The bank was helpful; her office was readied for patients.

She came in to her office every morning on the clanging little trolley that clicked and clacked its way between Stroudsburg and Delaware Water Gap, ending its brisk run at Seventh and Main Streets, to circle around the block and start its return trip. At first she took Bobby with her, and as her practice increased they trotted around town and into the hills with a horse and buggy rented from the town livery stable. By the end of three months she could pay her bills and she and Bobby could both eat well. One of Nina's new patients offered to keep Bobby during the day in exchange for doctoring for the entire family. The patient lived near Dr. Nina's office so Mother could stop in often to see that all was well. When her afternoon office hours were over, she picked up the child and clicked and swayed back to Delaware Water Gap on the busy little trolley.

I wonder why we gave up trolleys. It seems to me incredible that we threw away, all at once, this economical, efficient means of public transportation. Trolleys were great. They were sometimes uncomfortable, but so are public buses, even with expensive and wasteful frills added. Trolleys moved with real authority; they clanged; the sound of the metal wheels on the metal tracks brought immediate respect; the shining tracks were fixed in place so that when a trolley came careening down the street, everybody else moved aside. Trolleys made no fumes. They carried the nomad urban public efficiently from one place to another, which is all one can ask from a vehicle of transportation.

They did an honest job of work. How could we have been so feckless as to throw them away? The trolleys that Washington, D.C., disposed of in 1962 now are clanging around the streets of Sarajevo in Yugoslavia, scattering peasants, animals, cars, bicyclists, and smiling young girls who wave gaily at the placid passengers being moved with dispatch to where they want to go. I wish we could have them back. In Sarajevo, they're not called trolleys or trams. They're called Washingtonies.

Long letters from Charles were being forwarded from Philadelphia. He described the country he was currently touring, the towns and cities, food, clothing, and customs. He suggested that Nina use the letters as a basis for writing a series of lectures for the tour he planned after his return. He never told her where she might reach him; he never asked how she was or how things were going for her. There was never a personal word. Nina was too occupied making a living ever to write the lectures.

Charles came back in April of 1913. He was annoyed that the lecture series had not been written, but there was now a new detachment in his attitude to Dr. Nina. Somewhere inside he had sailed away from her. She must have known he was gone; all of us know when a close friend suddenly becomes an indifferent stranger. A bell tolls in the heart—gone! gone!—before the reluctant mind accepts the already felt loss. But Nina wasn't one to accept defeat easily. Almost six more years of trying were to pass before she acknowledged that he never, never would love her, although she attracted love from all other directions.

I can surmise all this with confidence because, in the notes and reminiscences about her first husband, she wipes out the next five-plus years—wipes them out with a bold, sturdy stroke. She recounts her disillusionment, her growing distaste for this man, her awareness that he was a poor bargain she could no longer accept. She rents an apartment in Stroudsburg, moves her furniture, her child, and her office into it, files for divorce. By the end of 1913 she is free and able to start a new life.

Except that it didn't happen that way. She didn't leave Charles until the winter of 1919, and she didn't divorce him until 1923. In the meantime, they had two more children, both girls, my sister Carol and me. When she wiped out those five-plus years, she wiped us out, too. It's eerie for us, and yet I can understand why, in her notes about her first marriage, we do not exist. When she wrote them, many years later but before Charles had died, she was looking back in bitterness and anger at his detachment, his rejection of her in 1913. How could she possibly explain two more children? She couldn't, so she didn't. It is, perhaps, a measure of the amount of emotion she had invested in their marriage that she could hate him so much for so long. The mirror image, the antimatter of one deep emotion is its opposite. It was not until he died before he was sixty years old that she forgave him for not loving her and was through with him. "A wind that passeth away, and cometh not again."

In fairness to my natural father, Charles couldn't have been all that dreadful. He too was trapped in a bad bargain. That he made the bargain when he was of an age to be wiser than he was is unimportant; wisdom arrives for each of us in its own time, and sometimes never comes at all. He reinforced his emotional detachment by a physical removal to answer a church call to become the preacher for a church in Parkersburg, West Virginia. It is interesting to find that his second wife, with whom, as far as I know, he lived a calm and happy life, came from there. Do you suppose they met then, in 1913? This would explain why Dr. Nina should suddenly, in May of 1914, leave her growing practice in Stroudsburg, pack her child and her belongings, and move in with Charles in West Virginia. Such a move seems incomprehensible, but the reasons for it may be very simple. Mother was not one to give up trying to achieve what was important to her. She may have decided to try again. She never mentions West Virginia in her notes, but fortunately there is external documentation and there are my memories of the West Virginia episode told to us as children.

She arrived in Parkersburg on May 13, and the next day she took the state medical examination to be licensed to practice medicine in West Virginia. She had no time to study or to worry about lack of preparation. A medical emergency existed in that area, and a special process had been created to license doctors from other states as quickly as possible. The examination started at eight in the morning and was to end at six in the afternoon.

The last hour of the examination was in a laboratory. Each doctor candidate was given a test tube full of urine and all the equipment necessary to test the specimen to determine the disease of the patient. All the doctors set out busily, some on one test, some on others, to isolate the patient's problem. All except Dr. Nina. She sat quietly at her lab station and concentrated on the specimen itself. Her clear, light-blue eyes were fixed with such intensity that she seemed to be breaking the fluid up into its components by willpower. It was this quality of intense concentration that, applied to her patients, made her a noted diagnostician. She looked and listened with her whole mind, and her patients, flattered and disconcerted by such close attention, went beyond a recital of large symptoms and added little seemingly unimportant details, one or more of which often gave Dr. Nina's trained, concentrated mind a clue to the real problem.

A faint warning light in the back of her mind was flashing. The specimen didn't look right to her. It didn't smell right. There was something queer about the specimen itself. She put her finger in the test tube and then in her mouth; she glanced up to see the doctor who was monitoring the examination looking at her with a big, bright grin and laughing eyes. She smiled back and wrote on her test paper: "If this is a urine specimen, the patient came from some other world. The specimen is water, sugar, and a coloring agent, and no one yet has died of it." She signed her paper and left. She was notified the next day that a license to practice medicine in West Virginia had been granted, and she joined the local doctors to help with the medical emergency.

What had come upon Wheeling, Parkersburg, and the little town of Fairmont, West Virginia, was the first outbreak of what, four and a half years later, was to sweep through our country the way smallpox swept through Europe and measles through Africa and the South Seas: the Great Flu Epidemic. Why first in West Virginia? Who brought it there in 1914? It is fortunate that deep in the hills travel was hard. The disease was confined because few people came or left. For Dr. Nina it was a valuable experience; she not only treated patients ill with the virus, but saw firsthand the complications that developed after the disease had run its course—the pneumonia, the lung abscesses, the empyema that finished off more patients than the influenza itself, and, where life continued, were to cause additional complications years and years later.

...5

For the period from the end of 1914 until summer of 1917 there are no written notes. Dr. Nina returned to Stroudsburg, and Charles, at some unknown time, answered a call to preach in a town in New Jersey. Dr. Nina had another baby, my sister Carol, in the Women's Medical College Pavilion Hospital in Philadelphia. She resumed her practice in Stroudsburg at her old office in the Stroudsburg *Daily Record* newspaper building on North Seventh Street, just down from the courthouse and just off Main Street. She and the children again lived on the mountain above Delaware Water Gap. Charles came at infrequent intervals, often bringing church people with him from New Jersey and Philadelphia, for whom Dr. Nina had to provide beds and meals.

It was in the early summer of 1917 that a new dimension was added to her medical practice. She began the medical care of one of the wildest, strangest, and wariest of all the deprived, neglected, and exclusive minority groups then known in the United States—Pennsylvania mountaineers who clustered in tiny settlements in the Poconos, far back in the hills where no one not of their own was allowed to come.

There were nine or ten little settlements of houses, each group a scattering of shacks, some within hollering distance from each other, in the solitude of trees at Brushy Mountain, Sal's Crotch, Skunk's Misery, Long Pond, Wildcat Hollow, and other then remote regions whose names are lost to me now. The inhabitants were remains of the great lumber camps that swept through the Appalachian

Mountains in the last years of the nineteenth century. The vigorous lumbermen swept on to western Pennsylvania, Ohio, Tennessee, but the weak ones, the shiftless, the misfits, the tired, and the gentle stayed behind, the second growth of trees sheltering them and the wild animals they needed for food. Their groupings were off the wagon trails. There was no visible way of communication between them, but they communicated. Warnings of danger, news of disasters, notices of shad runs and movements of deer herds flashed from group to group, no one ever knew how. The women who stayed with the lumbermen were camp followers. Among them all, even at the beginning, there was scarcely one tradition, scarcely a single set of moral values upon which a cultural community life could be constructed. Unlike the Virginia and Kentucky mountaineers, they started out with nothing of background or character and went on, by themselves, from there. Their marriages were by common law, but as moral precepts, never embedded, paled from generation to generation, intercourse was frequent between family members; mothers had sons by their sons, fathers by daughters, sisters by brothers. A wild, wooly, hairy, malformed, often idiot, sometimes brilliant clientele, and, to anyone who was fortunate enough to listen to Dr. Nina's stories about her fifteen-year care and service to them, hilariously funny and wonderfully, beautifully touching.

They're all gone now, the best of the children absorbed into our everyday American life. The outside world started buying motor cars and demanding roads to drive them on. Progress was ruthless in cutting between and into and over their wilderness homes. What revenue agents and truant officers and health authorities, cowards all, failed to do, Henry Ford and mass production accomplished without bloodshed. But the shades of our Pocono mountaineers, flickering like Indians among the dappled trees along the highways, should not be entirely forgotten. They fought the intrusion of an alien world upon their solitude with courage and perseverance and they lost the battle, maybe the last battle ever fought in the East against the Industrial Revolution. And they adopted Dr. Nina as their own and trusted her forever.

One summer afternoon Dr. Nina was packing her medical bag to start out on her round of home visits when she heard someone enter the waiting room. The man standing by the entrance door was tall and lean, and his long, lank hair hung down to his shoulders. His clothes were scarecrow rags. The skin of his face was creased and folded and burned to the color and texture of cowhide that had been exposed on a barn door to sun and wind. His eyes were narrow, deep-set. There was a strange tension about his body, so that for a moment Dr. Nina wondered if, should she say the wrong thing, he would leap upon her, or if he would leap back out of the half-opened door. He seemed poised for violent movement.

"Be ye the woman doctor?" he asked. Dr. Nina said that she was. "Tommy Allen, back to Wildcat Holler, is sick for days," he said, " 'n today he's struck with death. His ma's carryin' on an' wants for you to come. Kin you come?"

For a moment Dr. Nina hesitated. The resentment of these mountain people against any trespassing by strangers near their cabins was legendary. In times past, dead bodies had been brought into town—a luckless truant officer, a revenuer, a city hunter who had wandered too close to those who shot at strangers. But she hesitated only for a moment.

"Yes, I'll come. What seems to be the matter with Tommy, and how old is he?" she asked.

"He's six, or thereabouts," the man answered. "I don't

rightly know what he's ailin' with. He smothers and chokes and has screamin' pains in his belly."

Dr. Nina's little mare was happy to trot out of town and down the country roads. As they penetrated deeper into the hills, the woods made the horse uneasy, but, soothed by the doctor's voice, she trotted briskly. By the time evening was drawing in, they were at Wildcat Hollow. There the mountaineer, who had not spoken a word the whole long way, tied the little mare to a tree. Dr. Nina lifted the front latch and went into the one-room cabin. She need not have been fearful of her reception. They were glad to see her— the mother, the father, and two other half-grown sons. The mountaineer who had fetched the doctor came in and latched the door behind him.

"It's good a you to come, Doc," the mother said. "Tommy's awful bad. Kin you help him?"

Tommy was on a pallet on the floor. Dr. Nina had the two men and the two boys, one at each corner of the blanket on which he lay, gently lift the child to a table where she could examine him. Tommy was very sick indeed. His skin, hot with fever, was drawn over his cheeks and forehead until it shone white with suffering. His eyes were too bright, and his black hair was matted with the sweat of pain. His breath smelled of infection. The shadow of death was on him. Dr. Nina's heart almost stood still as she examined his distended abdomen. There was no doubt—a ruptured appendix. What should I do? she thought to herself. He's too near death, it's too late to take him twenty miles to the hospital. There isn't time to send for help. What can be done? There might be a chance, she thought, if I dared to open up his abdomen. How can I persuade his folks, these strange, dark, hairy creatures, to let me try? She searched her mind for a way to explain to them what the problem was, and what she proposed to do. She motioned

them to gather around and she drew on the back of a prescription blank a picture of Tommy's insides, demonstrat-
ing by pointing to his swollen stomach. She showed them
her surgery kit and the knife she proposed to use. She
showed them where she would make the incision and told
them what they could expect to happen. She was surprised
that they understood both the need for the immediate operation and its risk.

"Go on, Doc," said the mother.

"Cut," said the father. "Do what ye kin."

Then she really was frightened. All the surgery she had
done since she left Melrose, Massachusetts, was obstetrical
surgery. What if she couldn't find the right place? What
should she do about anesthetics? If she gave none, the physical shock might kill the child. If she gave ether, which was
all she had with her, he might drift all the way into death
with its fumes. She had time to be thoroughly frightened
while her instruments were boiling.

If he dies, she thought, they will never let me out of here
alive. Suddenly she was ashamed. Why was she thinking of
herself when it was for such a moment as this that she had
become a doctor? She was ashamed, and shame banished
panic. As she waited for the handle of the surgical knife to
cool, she leaned over the suffering child.

"Tommy," she said, "I'm going to help you feel better,
but you must do what I tell you. Put this wad of gauze
between your front teeth. I'm going to put more gauze over
your nose and mouth and drip some cold, smelly stuff on
it. You must breathe deeply, and some of the pain will go
away. You must look straight into my eyes. When I tell you
to, bite hard on the gauze in your mouth and close your
eyes. Then *don't move*, no matter what. Are you ready?"

The child nodded, his eyes wild with sickness and fright.
Dr. Nina dripped ether slowly on the gauze, just enough

until the brightness in his eyes began to dim and the wildness to fade. She removed the ether gauze, signaled to the father and the neighbor to hold the child still, said, "Tommy! Close your eyes and bite hard!" and, to herself, God help me, and cut into his body. Tommy gave one scream and fainted. Pus poured out. Dr. Nina worked fast. She didn't try to remove the appendix. She put in a large gauze drain and strapped a light dressing firmly over the incision. They lowered Tommy back on his pallet. Dr. Nina sat on a chair and watched him by lantern light throughout the night, changing the dressing often. She was encouraged when three o'clock came and went, and four, and five, those hours in which the grievously afflicted are most apt to stop fighting death. By sunup, her trained eyes detected a faint improvement. His forehead and cheekbones were less glisteningly white, his moans were softer and less fitful, his pulse was stronger. She packed her doctor's bag, left instructions to be followed until she returned later in the day, untied her little mare, and, as soon as they were out of the deep woods, tied the reins to the buckboard, stretched out on the buggy seat, and slept, while the little brown mare delicately and soberly chose all the right roads home.

Wherever Dr. Nina went that morning for house calls, she asked for help for Tommy. By midafternoon the buggy was loaded with eggs, meat for broth, canned milk, preserves; and on the seat beside the doctor was Daisy, a nanny goat, her long legs folded up neatly under her as she gazed at the countryside, enjoying her outing.

Daisy was a pet goat that had been given to Dr. Nina by a farm family in payment for the delivery of twins. She furnished milk for the doctor's children, and endless amusement. Her favorite pastime was to fold herself neatly on one seat of the lawn swing and, by moving her head back and forth, set herself swinging slowly while she chewed her cud. She followed everyone going up and down the road until one day, when a family had gone to the station to watch the daily train puff and billow into the station and blow and wheeze its way out, Daisy had eaten all the labels off the trunks unloaded from the train. Since then, she had been enclosed.

Tommy was noticeably better. His incision still was draining, but now it was a light, odorless fluid that had a healthy look. His temperature was down. It was obvious that death had been put to flight. He fell in love with Daisy on sight, and Daisy with Tommy. She folded herself neatly on a bench against the wall near Tommy's pallet and there she stayed, smiling her foolish goat grin, except when she went outside to eat the tender ferns or to be milked. Dr. Nina took Daisy home after Tommy was well, but Daisy had been spoiled for outdoor life. All night long she pounded with her hoofs on the door to be allowed to come in. With the doctor's next trip into the mountains, Daisy went back to where, neatly folded, she could share the lives of five people who lived and bickered, bore and forbore, and cared for each other and for her, all in a one-room shack deep in the woods where strangers were not allowed.

This was in 1917, before Dr. Nina bought her first Ford car. In 1964, this little story had a sequel in which I was involved. When Mother closed her office to devote her time to her ailing ninety-two-year-old second husband, those of us who could came to take turns staying in the office to tell unnotified or unnoticing patients that Dr. Nina was no longer in practice.

One morning when I was on duty, I heard the waiting-room door open and close. I found a man sitting on the couch. He was dressed in a trucker's uniform with the name of a moving and hauling firm on his cap. He was a big man, burly, a little overweight, but strong-looking and healthy. He appeared to be somewhere in his fifties.

"I come for some pills for the missus," he said. "The doc give her some five years ago that done fine. Now she's got the same complaint and wants some more pills. Just tell the doc it's for Mrs. Transit. Doc Nina will know what pills."

When I told him the doctor wasn't doctoring any more, he jumped to his feet, his face red and his big hands curled into fists.

"She can't do this to us!" he shouted. "She saved my life when I was a boy. She cut me open on a table and saved my life. She's taken care of us all—my missus, the kids. She can't do this to us!"

I said I was sorry. He stood for a moment, the red fading from his face. Then he spread out his big hands, palms up, in a most appealing and pathetic gesture, and, looking straight into my face, asked softly, "What will become of us now?"

At dinner that night I told the story of Mr. Transit in the office. Mother told about Tommy, and what made Tommy Transit so important. He was her first case back in the woods with the mountaineers. After Tommy's operation, word spread like a grass fire through the hills. "That woman doc's all right. She'll come if ye need 'er. She kin help ye. She'll take what ye have to give 'er fur pay, and if ye don't got nothin' to give, she'll come anyway." More and more calls came from telephones in lonely general stores, notes were brought and put in her mailbox by shy, wild creatures who slipped into town and slipped quickly out. Wherever and whenever she was needed, she went. And they trusted her.

One time, when she was washing and dressing a newborn baby in clothes she had brought with her, she heard a neighbor, passing by the Brushy Mountain cabin, say to the baby's father, "Doc Nina's all right! There ain't nary a one of us in the hills wouldn't wipe her ass for her if she needed it."

After Tommy's operation Dr. Nina's medical care of the mountaineers brought a bright new dimension into the lives of them all.

...6

And then came the winter of despair, the dreadful winter, the winter of 1918. Dr. Nina had had a rewarding summer. Some of the men doctors had gone to war, although most were over draft age. Her income had grown modestly because, in order to survive at all as a doctor, she had to set her fees pitifully low in comparison to those charged by men. One dollar for an office visit, two for a home visit, medicine always included, and $25 for delivering a baby. Charles had come to visit in the spring and Dr. Nina was again pregnant. By Armistice time, in November, she had stocked the pantry full of food for the winter, had had a modest supply of wood stacked near the house, had arranged for Bobby and Carol to stay with Mrs. Kotz, and in due time had gone to Philadelphia to birth her baby, who was me. Having a baby, by then, was no big deal for Dr. Nina. She was back in ten days, picked up her other two girls, and moved into the house on the hill. Then came the snow.

Snow came upon snow, with the only pauses days of slashing wind and sleet and ice storms. No days of thaw, only snow piling on snow and ice. The temperature reached and held at an astonishing low for that section of the country. The world of the Poconos was immobilized in snow.

The house that Charles had designed was odd. It was

square and low to the ground. It was made of cobblestones that jutted out from the cement that held them together. The front porch, cement, was wide, with a brown wood-shingled roof with eaves that came deep in front toward the ground, a cool, shaded porch looking out over the valley below. The front door opened directly into the living room, a large square windowless room with seven doors opening from it, and a huge, walk-in fireplace made of cobblestones at the far end. There were two doors on either side of the fireplace, one to the kitchen with a big iron stove, a sink with a hand pump, and an icebox, the other to a storage and laundry room with two big galvanized iron tubs and a narrow door into the kitchen so that hot water could be carried from the wood-burning stove. The other four doors, two on either side of the big square living room, opened into four small bedrooms. There were windows in the bedrooms, but the eaves of the low-pitched, raftered roof came close to the ground and light from the windows was pale, watery, diffuse. Even in summer with all the doors open, the living room was dark; in winter it was perpetual night, the light from the fireplace and kerosene lamps lost in the dark shadows. I don't know what this house tells us about the man who designed it. Surely it must make a statement about Charles. That his imprecise mind was relaxed and comfortable only away from the light of facts? That he was so self-centered that only a cave could reflect his own nature? Surely a house one creates for oneself tells something important about the designer. The house had no central heating. I suspect that Charles did not intend to live there in the winters himself.

But Dr. Nina and the children were there when the snow and the biting cold descended upon them. She hadn't worried about wood for the fireplace or the stove. The year before, a small lumber company had set up a camp beyond the house and above Cherry Valley on the other side of the mountain. The crew was small and worked the year round. They carried their second-growth logs down to the railroad in Delaware Water Gap every two weeks, in summer in drays and in winter in sledges. The men were willing to saw, split, and drop off firewood for the houses along the way. Dr. Nina had counted on the lumbermen. None of them had counted on being immobilized for more than a month over Christmas and the New Year of 1919, and the lumber camp burned its own wood and went on half rations and swore roundly at the snow that kept the men away over the holidays from those they loved and were working for.

The cold was so intense that most of Dr. Nina's wood was burned by Christmas. She was not in good health. I know this because four years later, at the divorce hearing, Mame McNeal testified that when Nina fled to her in mid-January at the nadir of her life and the debacle of her marriage, she was "in miserable health." I know this because another wonderful woman, Emma Fargo, a neighbor more than a mile down the hill toward Delaware Water Gap, testified in the same legal proceeding that she and her husband, worried about little Dr. Nina, forced their way up on foot just after the New Year, to make sure Nina was all right, alone as she was with three little children in the worst of a bad winter. Halfway up the hill, Mr. Fargo had to turn back; he had had a mild heart attack a year before and couldn't exert himself physically any further. Mrs. Fargo was struggling through the deep snow wrapped in a long racoon coat. She gave her coat to Mr. Fargo to take back home; she could not maneuver the bottom of the coat through the drifts. She still had on several layers of warm wool sweaters. Two hours later, a veritable snow woman, she reached her goal.

At the house she found the children's beds pulled out into the living room and set up near the fireplace. A small fitful fire burned in the giant fireplace. The room was barely above freezing. The children were kept in bed to keep them warm. Dr. Nina had chopped down the trees near the house that were small enough for her to handle, but they had burned too quickly to give much heat. In desperation she had forced her way through the drifts to the boundary of a neighbor's property and dragged back his fence rails. Emma Fargo stated in court: "Little Dr. Nina, the best wife and mother in the whole world, was white as paper and thin as air."

The doctor must have been frightened each time she pushed her way out over the drifted porch and plunged into the deep, ever falling snow, struggling to keep her footing on the ice beneath. If something happened to her, if she couldn't get back, the children would surely freeze to death. How thankful she must have been each time she reached the safety of the porch again, dragging behind her as many stolen fence rails as she could pull! She sawed them up on the porch, her hands numb with cold. No wonder she was white as paper and thin as air.

On the tenth of January the snow stopped falling. The skies cleared. The temperature, in the strange way it often does on the eastern seaboard in January, rose and rose and rose. The snow and ice melted in cascades down the mountain slopes, the Delaware River rose beyond flood stage, and the forsythia, that zany spring-flowering shrub that can be fooled any time by any deception of nature, pushed out fat yellow buds.

Mr. Bartron, the neighboring farmer, took a tour around his barns and fields to assess the bad-weather damage to his place. He found a large section of his rail fence missing from the field closest to "that preacher's" house. He had chopped down the trees and split the rails himself in his youth to build a fence that was to last longer than his own life. He was struck with fury to find them gone. Rage boiling within carried him heavily but swiftly to the neighbor's house. He shouted at the front door, open to let in sun and warmth, and he met Dr. Nina in the middle of the dim living room as she hurried out of the kitchen, startled by the noise. He told her at length what he thought of pretend-Christians who would steal from others.

Nina sat down on a chair and listened until he had said everything he could think of to say. Then she said, "I'm sorry—I was alone. The lumbermen didn't come and there was no place else to get wood. I'll have them replaced when I can work again to pay for them. I couldn't let my children freeze. I was sick at heart to take them, but there was nothing else to do." She tried to say more, but her voice quavered. She bowed her head. Fat tears splashed down on her hands folded in her lap.

Mr. Bartron was silent. All his rage drained away. The tiny fence-rail fire in the big fireplace hissed quietly; the faint voices of children outside in the sun carried through the open door.

"I'm the one that's sorry," he said. "We didn't know you was all alone here, but we should have knowed. We should have come to see. We thought we was good neighbors, but we've been bad neighbors to you. Come, lass, don't cry. I thought on the way here," he added wonderingly, "that I'd sue you for taking my fence. Now I'd be glad if you'd sue me. It would make me feel better. If you'll forgive me for not helping, we'll never talk of this again." He patted her awkwardly on the shoulder and left. Before nightfall he and two of his sons were back with a wagonload of fireplace wood and stovewood from the lumber camp.

On the fifteenth of January, winter came back. The forsythia froze, but inside the cavelike house fire roared in the fireplace and the big iron range in the kitchen glowed iron-red under the cook pots. On that day Charles arrived in time for supper. He had come for a purpose, but for the wrong purpose at the wrong time. He had, he said, decided to build a new sanitarium, and he'd come to find out how much money Nina had saved from her summer's work.

"You surely must have some money saved up. I have a chance to buy some electrical equipment secondhand but in wonderful condition, as good as new, for about one-fourth its original cost. With what money you have, and what we can get for selling your office equipment, we can buy it."

Perhaps the snow and ice of the month-long blizzard had been left, unthawed, in Nina's heart.

"I have nothing saved that you can have."

"What! Nothing saved? I don't believe you! You're lying. What have you done with all the money you've made?" Charles was shouting now.

"I've paid the hospital bills and the doctor for my confinement. I've paid back the loan at the bank and a loan from friends. I've bought food for the winter. I've bought furniture for this house. I have no money for you. What little I have left is for the children."

Charles was beside himself with anger. "I married you because I'd heard how smart you were! I thought you'd be a great success as a doctor. But you've disappointed me in every way. You've disgraced yourself and lost your influence with the church. You've persisted in the crazy idea of having children. You take care of disgusting mountain sinners without pay. You're a wicked woman! You don't know your place!"

The phone rang.

The Reverend Crown, the Methodist minister in the town of Portland, Pennsylvania, at the other end of the trolley line from Stroudsburg, was calling to see if Dr. Nina could come. His mother-in-law was feeling poorly. I now quote from the divorce proceedings later:

Answer [Dr. Nina]: The telephone rang and Reverend Crown wanted me to come to see his wife's mother. I told him I could not come, I was not able to go out. I told him if they could not get another doctor, I would come in the morning. I had supper to get for my children; I had been doing a big wash all day and was physically unable to come. The weather was nasty and I would have had to walk down to the Gap to get the trolley and then walk back from the trolley home in the dark. That's how the fuss started.

"Fuss" is a mild word for what happened next. Charles lost all control. "You don't want to help!" he shouted, and physically attacked Nina.

How could this be? Such a thing doesn't happen to people we know. Or does it? And is a physical attack worse or better than a verbal attack that demolishes every hope and every dream? If neither proves to be fatal, if either ends a losing game, I suppose it's a toss-up between them as to which form of retaliation brings to a close a part of one's life that began in error and must end, as all important errors do, in direct or subtle violence.

Surely an act of violence by a minister whose gospel was peace and love was not brought on by any real concern for electrical equipment, even though electricity then had a glamour and excitement we would scarcely believe today, or by the loss of a two-dollar house-call fee. Whatever caused Charles to explode is forever hidden in his frustrations, thwarted ambitions, and secret fears.

But that this should happen to Dr. Nina, after all her valiant efforts to create out of nothing a life worth living, angers me all these years later. I lose my detachment, I become involved, raised as I was, as we all were, on the great Cinderella myth, which promises that if we are good and hard-working and patient and uncomplaining, and are also very, very pretty, then a prince will come, dressed all in pale-blue satin, and he will ask, "Will you marry me?" and we will all live happily ever after.

Thin-as-air Dr. Nina was good, hard-working, patient, and uncomplaining. She was also stalwart, capable to stand, braver than the panthers that lurked along her way. She was very pretty. And her clerical-collared prince knocked her down, flung himself upon her under the eyes of their children, and tried to squeeze her life out of her slender throat. She was saved by little Bobby, who grabbed her father's hair and shrieked into his ear until he regained emotional control before Dr. Nina was totally dead. Pale and shaken himself, he took his unopened valise and left.

How could it come to this, the courage, the fortitude, the merry heart? Was God distracted, watching some sparrow fall in a faraway place? Is this the fulfillment of the promise that all will be well with the righteous, this slight, thin-as-air form unconscious on the floor of a cavelike room? Wept over only by a desolate child? "These tears are shaken from the wrath-bearing tree."

...7

Dr. Nina's injuries were temporary; one small bone broken in her throat and her vocal cords temporarily paralyzed. She was able to reassure Bobby, give the children their supper and their baths, and put them to bed that night without fear of further misfortune. They imitated mother in whispering, which was all the noise Nina would be able to make for the next three weeks. She packed all their clothes and, in the morning, after putting the suitcases on the front porch, carried two children, with Bobby trailing along, into Delaware Water Gap. She arranged for someone to pick up the suitcases later in the day and to put them on the last trolley run in the evening. She and the children boarded the trolley and went to Stroudsburg, to Mame McNeal. The following day she went to a throat specialist in Philadelphia. The day after that, back in Stroudsburg, she rented an apartment on Main Street, on the second floor above a men's and boys' clothing store. The steep, narrow staircase up to the apartment was between the clothing store and a drugstore that is still in the same location. She hired men to bring the furniture from the Delaware Water Gap house and the office equipment from her office around the corner on Seventh Street into the new apartment. When everything was in place, she and her children moved in. And so, all in whispers, she was ready to begin a new era.

As often happens when one takes decisive action to end past mistakes and begin again, new doors to the future opened of themselves. Two unexpected events were to make Dr. Nina's immediate future less uncertain: Anne Barr arrived out of a cold, dark night, and a virulent epidemic of influenza broke out in the area as part of the Great Flu Epidemic of 1918–19.

The apartment was a "flat" in the British sense of the word. At the top of the long, steep stairway from Main Street there was a landing with two doors, one to the right, which entered into the front room, and one straight ahead, which led into a long, narrow, windowless hallway that ran the length of the flat and ended at a landing for the steep back stairs and the kitchen. The hallway was designed to furnish privacy for the three bedrooms that opened from it, but the little family needed reassurance and togetherness more than privacy, so the hallway was used for storage and the door kept locked. The front room had a bay window overlooking Main Street, and a cunning coal-burning fireplace; this was to be the waiting room for Dr. Nina's patients. The next room back was to be her office. The office and the three bedrooms behind it were windowless, but each had a skylight in the ceiling. Skylights are wonderful. One can lie in bed and watch the moon racing through the clouds, or the brilliant winter stars still and cold in the endless velvety universe, or, at early morning, a heedless bird who has plunged into solid glass and shakes his witless head to wonder, no doubt, whose hand has struck him down. To reach the kitchen from the front room, one walked through all the succeeding rooms. The rent, the first two months, was $18 a month, but the shocking inflation that followed the end of the First World War soon boosted it to $28 a month. The rent included heat from a coal furnace in the basement. The handyman from the clothing store tended the furnace during the day, and after five o'clock banked the furnace for the night. By the time the flat became chilled, the children were in bed, office hours were over, and Dr. Nina could sit by a cozy coal fire in the front room. Nina and the baby shared the first bedroom, Bobby and Carol the second, and the bedroom next to the big, bright kitchen was reserved, unknown to everyone until the second evening of their residence, for Anne Barr.

Anne Barr was seventeen, pregnant, and desolate when she came to the waiting-room door that night. Her mother was dead, her father had decamped for parts unknown, the father of her baby had been killed in the war the day before the Armistice. Hungry and alone, she could think of nothing else to do to save herself but to walk almost twenty miles to ask help from the "woman doctor." She was to live with Dr. Nina for three years. She was to flourish. She did lessons at night with Bobby, who was already in the fourth grade; she learned to cook; she became an expert seamstress and made clothes for all the children, including her own fat, rosy baby girl. She was as happy as a domestic kitten and as friendly and winning. After three years she left the household to marry a young printer who worked at a local printing plant. They lived happily ever after, as far as I know. For Dr. Nina she was a godsend. Now Nina could take on any case, any time, day or night, because there would always be someone there to watch the children. Anne truly liked children; we were her best friends and we were very happy together.

The second event, the flu epidemic, hit all at once all over town. The armed services held the younger doctors long after the war was finished. The older doctors took turns catching the virus. All who could stand on their feet worked day and night. The hospitals overflowed into hotels; volunteer workers helped tend the sick and bury the dead. Soup wagons went from door to door. Dr. Nina caught nothing and was the busiest doctor of all.

As the epidemic slowed in the town, calls began to pour in from the farms and the mountains. Few of the men doctors would go on these calls. Two of them owned Ford cars, but even in good weather they refused to risk their new toys on the wretched back roads. That year the roads were blocked with snow and ice. Anyway, the fees charged by the men doctors were too high for this new group of stricken citizenry. Dr. Nina finally had to ask the county medical officer for help. He found a sleigh for her, manned by volunteer drivers, with two teams of horses, two horses for day and two for night. Her volunteer drivers changed every twelve hours with the fresh horses. Nina slept in the sleigh between houses. The ladies' aid societies and the missionary societies of various churches took turns making large vats of soup from meat donated by the butchers of the town. The soup, and oranges and eggs wrapped to keep them from freezing, filled the sleigh on every trip.

When the drivers came to a road that branched off from the main road toward a house, they drove in to ask if anyone were sick. Often the entire family was afflicted, with no one to cook. While the drivers brought in wood and built up fires, Dr. Nina fixed medicine and food. Then on they went to the next place. They soon learned to recognize that where no path had been broken up the lane to a house or cabin, conditions inside were apt to be dreadful. One night, near morning, in a shack in the hills, they found a mother and daughter dead, a man having a hemorrhage, two older girls too sick to get up, and two small, wet, nearly frozen children huddled in a crib. It took some time to get that place in shape to leave, even temporarily.

When she was back in town to change horses and drivers, Dr. Nina persuaded the medical officer to wire Harrisburg to send a state nurse to help. One was sent immediately. At midnight the following night she was in the sleigh, looking with fear into the dark woods as they forced their way through new-fallen snow back to the shack. Nina tried to encourage her when she left her in charge.

"Just do the best you can. Feed the two little ones. Keep the fire going. Force liquids—soup or fruit juice, it doesn't matter—into the sick. We'll be back about this time tomorrow night. There's enough medicine 'til then."

When Dr. Nina came back the next night, Miss Milnor, the nurse, could hardly talk for tears.

"What's the matter? Are you ill? Your patients are all much better and the place looks wonderful. Why are you crying?"

"I'm not ill. I'm hungry and I haven't had anything to drink since you left."

"Why didn't you eat? There's plenty of food in the house."

"I couldn't eat. They keep the food under the bed. And the dishes and pans—they're awful!"

"Well, there's plenty of water to drink."

"Yes, but I saw a horse drinking out of the spring!"

Nina had to suppress a laugh. "Don't worry about the horses. They're the cleanest things here. Besides, the spring cleans itself almost by the time an animal stops drinking. And I'll show you how to have a good meal, even here."

While a pail of water was heating, Nina scoured the pans and the coffeepot and pine-board table with ashes from the front of the stove and rinsed them all with boiling water. She sliced venison from under the bed, fried potatoes, and made coffee. They had a fine midnight meal.

Years later the nurse, on her way through Stroudsburg, stopped to reminisce with Dr. Nina.

"Doctor," she said, "I learned the greatest lesson of my life in the woods with you. Do you remember the men by the roadside who had come to shovel out drifts so we could get through that first night?"

"You mean the ones who had the bonfire and a pot of coffee waiting for us?"

"Yes. I was horrified when I saw you drink coffee from that tin can. And you thanked them for it! One of the men said, 'We thought you'd be cold and tired, and coffee kinda springs you up, don't it?' You said, 'It sure does, Joe.' I thought, The doctor says that exactly as though she means it, and then I found out you really did mean it! I was disgusted. What kind of doctor is this? I asked you how you could drink out of a dirty can that maybe the man had been drinking out of and you laughed and said, 'You know, nurse, one of my patients told me that everyone eats a peck of dirt before he dies. I think this was the time for me to eat a little of mine. These men walked miles and worked hours to open the road for us. I wouldn't have refused to drink their coffee if it had been twice as black and dirty!' Then you shut your eyes and went to sleep.

"All these years since, when something hard or disagreeable comes up, I think of you and wonder what you would do, and I've always found a way out."

...8

Dr. Nina earned more money in her twenty-four-hours-a-day service during the flu epidemic than she'd ever earned before, and it was all hers. She also had acquired many new patients who would depend upon her and whose children and grandchildren would depend upon her until she closed her practice at the age of eighty-two.

She took $475 of her nest egg and bought a Model T Ford. A fellow townsman had purchased the car in Philadelphia, had driven it to Stroudsburg on what was, for him, a terrifying journey, vowed never to touch a horseless carriage again, and unloaded it on "that woman doctor." And so began a most perfect union, the union between Dr. Nina and a series of machines that were to liberate her from the tyranny of large animals and that were to enable her to practice her profession in exactly the way she dreamed it could be done. She could go wherever she was needed by making outrageous demands on metal that she would not have dared to make on any living thing.

She was respectful of the motor of each of her automobiles, her "pleasure cars," as all motor vehicles that were not trucks were called in the early days. Engines were semihuman. They needed food and water and understanding. In those days, car-engine mechanisms were almost as easy for an ordinary owner to comprehend as a sewing-machine motor. But she made the assumption that the metal bodies could take their own chances in a hard world; wherever tender flesh and brittle bone wished to go, surely tough metal would manage to come along. So she mercilessly drove her cars over farm fields, through brush, brambles, and mountain berry bushes, over goat tracks and wagon trails, leaving a canvas top hanging from a low branch here and a piece of running board in a deep rut there, and a fender on a rock in a creek bed, until she was driving a stripped-down machine that any of the hot-rodders of the 1950s would have given their souls to own. At that point she would buy a new car.

She named her first car Donkey. The man she bought it from gave her driving instructions. He showed her where to place the spark handle and the manual accelerator handle before she started to crank at the front of the car; he showed her how to leap like a gazelle back to the gadgets to adjust them to keep the once-caught motor going, how to release the hand brake, which kept the transmission in neutral, how to depress the clutch to shift into low, and how to shift into high and sail away down the road. He forgot to tell her the car could back up. She found that out three weeks later from the husband of one of her patients who had watched with bewilderment as she sailed around his house, scattering chickens and geese and causing minor damage to his woodpile on one side and his corncrib on the other as she drove out forward from an impasse she had driven herself into forward. He flagged her down and explained that the middle foot pedal, when pushed in, would put the car into reverse. From then on, Donkey took her anywhere she intended to reach. When she cranked up her

Ford in the middle of the night to go to deliver a baby, the neighbors who briefly woke as she went rattlety-bang down Main Street must have thought, There goes the woman doctor! before they snuggled back into oblivion.

One evening she was on her way home down Brushy Mountain. It was cold and a misty drizzle had silently turned the deeply rutted, stony road into thick mud. Her Model T reared up on one side, came down with splashes and rattles, reared up over a stone on the other side, and stalled. She cranked and cranked; the car refused to start. Her patience was worn thin and her arms began to weaken when Donkey caught with a roar and bucked toward her in a vehement leap. Dr. Nina was the more practiced leaper, however, and her foot found the running board and her hand the steering wheel as Donkey bucked on by. Halfway down the mountain, the flaring headlights revealed a man slogging through the mud. Dr. Nina pulled up beside him.

"Going toward town?" she asked cheerfully. "Want a ride?"

"Be ye that woman doctor?" he asked.

"Yes, I am."

He shook his head. "Thank ye kindly jist the same, but I guess I'll walk."

Nina was astonished. "I won't hurt you," she said.

"I know. I hain't afeared of you, I'm afeared of your drivin'. They do tell that you'd drive through hell or the pearly gates to git whar you're goin'."

One February evening in 1920, during a winter thaw, Dr. Nina was driving as fast as she could go to Brown's Run, twenty-five miles from town. It was eleven o'clock at night. She was rushing to a child who was reported to be choking to death on something lodged in her throat. The child's father had walked five miles to the nearest phone.

She worried as she drove along because, to reach the shack, she would have to cross Bear Swamp. The road across the swamp was laid on logs and it was reasonably easy to follow in daylight, but at night, with the bog liquified by the thaw, she worried that she might slide off into the deep holes on either side and be hopelessly stuck. The problem was complicated by the fact that the lights of the Model T shone brightly at full speed, glowed dimly at a slow crawl over difficult terrain, and went off altogether when the motor stalled, as it often did after a good, solid jounce.

As she neared the swamp, she saw a lantern bobbing off in the woods, higher up than the road. She stopped the car and blew the horn. The light stood still. She blew again and then again, and the light began to bob down toward her. When the man who carried the lantern reached the car, he raised it up even with his face and peered into the car. Dr. Nina shrank back with fear. He looked like a gorilla. A bushy beard covered his entire face and his hair hung down on his shoulders. He grinned a big, wide grin and all the teeth he had were two tusks on either side of his mouth.

"Be ye that woman doctor?" he asked.

Thank God, thought Dr. Nina. At least it talks. She realized that he must be Old Featherhead, a hermit about whom there were many strange tales. One tale was told of a hunter who disappeared near Bear Swamp and had never been found. But Old Featherhead was glimpsed later wearing new hunting boots.

The doctor said, "Yes, I am. I blew the horn to ask you to go with me across the swamp, so that if I should get stuck, you could help me get out."

"Well," the old man rolled a big cud of tobacco over into his other cheek and spat a brown stream of juice over his shoulder, "I hain't never rid in one of these dang things, but I guess I kin, if you kin."

"Set your lantern in the back on the floor and get in the front with me."

Featherhead climbed in. He took a firm grip on the back of the seat with one hand and on the car door with the other, chewing fast on his quid. Why, thought the doctor, this poor man is more frightened of the car than I am of him! To ease his tension, she told him about the child.

"That must be Jim Walker's kid," he said.

Driving as fast as she could, she crossed the swamp and pulled into a clearing. Old Featherhead started to climb out with his lantern.

"Oh, please don't leave me!" exclaimed the doctor. "Maybe you can help. And I'll need you to get back out of here."

The old man stopped chewing his tobacco and looked at her strangely.

"You really want Old Featherhead to stay and help you?"

"Yes. Please do."

Just then the cabin door opened, and they went in together. The Walker cabin was larger than most. It had two rooms, both of good size. The front door opened into the kitchen–living room. Next to this room was a small bedroom, where the parents and two younger children slept. The three older children slept on cots close to the kitchen stove. None of the children were in bed; they waited forlornly for the doctor, anxiously watching their mother and the choking baby on her lap. The three-year-old's lips were blue; she was barely breathing in hoarse, rasping gasps. Her eyes were rolled back in her head.

Dr. Nina turned the child over on its stomach. While the mother held the baby's feet up so that the head was down, the doctor reached down the child's throat and her finger found a piece of raw potato so firmly lodged that it had shut off most of the air. Fortunately, the irregular shape of the obstruction had allowed enough air to be drawn in by the oxygen-famished lungs to keep the child alive, although she was cyanosed and unconscious.

After the obstruction was removed, the child turned from blue to white and, after a few moments of artificial respiration, pink, and began to howl. The mother cried with relief. The children vied with each other to play, all at the same time, the baby's favorite games to welcome her back to life. Into the scene of bedlam came the father after his ten-mile walk. He was as excited and relieved as everyone else.

"I didn't think you'd come yet, Doc," he said. "I didn't see no car tracks over the bridge in the swamp."

"We never come over no bridge!" announced Old Featherhead. All the noise stopped in surprise.

"How'd you git here, then?" Jim asked.

"Wal," and Old Featherhead paused to squirt an accurate brown stream of tobacco juice into the open draft door of the stove, sizzling the ashes, "we just jumped the clean hell over!"

Bedlam resumed, but now it was Dr. Nina who laughed the most. Old Featherhead couldn't have been more pleased with himself and with his joke. He glowed like an ember.

As Dr. Nina was packing her doctor's bag to leave, Jim spoke quietly.

"I can't pay you nothin' now, Doc, cause I ain't got nothin'. When they pay me for my work in the woods I'll bring somethin' in. O.K.?"

"That's all right. Pay me when you can," and she thought to herself, Promises, promises! They go on like the dead stumps in the swamp.

A few weeks later, as Dr. Nina came out of the hospital on the edge of town, she saw Old Featherhead leaving her car. He spied her and came back.

"Doc," he whispered, "I put somethin' in the back of your car for you. Eat it and keep your mouth shut."

In the car was a quarter of young, tender, out-of-season venison. From then on, she often found a pheasant or a box of trout packed in wet fern and moss or a rabbit on the floor in the rear of the car.

One day one of her mountaineer patients said, "Doc, what you done to Old Featherhead to make him like he be now?"

"Like he be now? Well, how is he?"

"Why, if your name come up in the talk, he says you is one of God's angels. He visits around, and lends a hand, and acts like a regular neighbor. He hain't never been like this since we can remember."

This pays my bill for the trip! the doctor thought.

...9

The intelligence apparatus among the mountaineers was amazing. Although miles separated them from each other, there was a grapevine network that moved as fast as ground fire to keep everyone informed of what was happening in their forest. Whenever a stranger set foot in their territory, everyone knew it. They resented outsiders not because they hated strange and different people but because the outsiders who came were sneering, critical, cold-eyed, and bossy. Except for their Dr. Nina, who was unfailingly courteous and respectful of their common humanity. Among themselves there was loyalty and trust; and the good things of their lives—the meat, the celebrations, the sorrows of honorable death—were shared among them all.

Old Lindy, a matriarch of a particularly isolated family, was preparing to die. At the most conservative estimate she was 105 years old. Her vital organs were worn out and faltering. Dr. Nina had urged her to stop drinking mountain dew, the home-distilled corn whiskey that was the only cash crop of the area.

"Your liver has all it can do without having to handle mountain dew," the doctor had told her.

"Jesus, Doc! Had I of knowed I'd live so long, I'd of took better care of my liver." Smiling a wide, toothless grin, her eyes snapping in glee, she poured a half cup from the jug by her bed and drank it down. Dr. Nina patted her shoulder. Old Lindy was right—it was too late for her to start a new life. The day Old Lindy died, Dr. Nina was called. Dozens of the forest people were there. The carcass of a young buck deer was roasting over a fire in the clearing in front of the two-room shack. Inside, the shack was full to bursting with neighbors. Dr. Nina confirmed that death had indeed taken Old Lindy. She sat down by the bed to fill out the death certificate. The man who had brought the funeral meat started to recount how he had shot the buck. Dr. Nina saw another man, a stranger to her, frantically motioning him to be quiet about out-of-season hunting.

"Aw, what's eatin' ye?" the first man asked. "Hell, Doc's one of us."

Dr. Nina pretended not to hear, but her heart rejoiced that there was no fear and distrust among them.

One night she was driving along a mountain road five miles back of Henryville. As she approached a narrow bridge across Bushkill Creek, she saw a light tiny as a firefly waving at the near end of the bridge. She pulled over to the side of the road as a man stepped out of the darkness, lighting another match and holding it high.

"Hello, Doc. I heared tell ye was comin' back to Hunters'

Range. My woman, up the creek, is bornin' our first young-
'un and she's powerful bad. It ain't fur from here. Will ye
come?"

"How do I get there?" Dr. Nina asked.

"We gotta walk. Leave the car here."

Dr. Nina got out with her bag and followed the hairy,
ragged man up a path almost closed by brush and briars. The man was a darker blotch ahead in the darkness
of the night. A little fear came into her mind. She wondered if there was really a house up such an unused
path. They came to the bank of Bushkill Creek and
climbed up some rocky steps to the beginning of a
bridge. It was a hanging footbridge made by stringing
two telephone wires across the noisy waters of the
gorge, with boards laid across the wires and a thin wire
on the side for a handrail.

"Hold on to me," the man said. "Walk slow so it don't
swing too much and we'll git over all right."

She could hear water rushing far below. Trembling a
little and clutching her medicine bag, she put her hand in
his and walked across the bridge in the dark, doing exactly
as he said. "Step wide here—a board's out. Stand still and
wait fer the bridge to stop swingin'. Here's the end—step
down deep."

The shack had one room and was dirty, bare, and cold.
She didn't know it then, but twenty years later, when the
baby she delivered that night was fighting in the Pacific in
the Second World War, Dr. Nina was to deliver his baby
to a pretty little wife in a neat little bungalow in Stroudsburg, a bungalow with running water, clean linen, and
handmade baby clothes lovingly laid out on a brand-new
bathinette. There was also a money order sent from
Okinawa for $100, and a note:

Dear Dr. Nina,

I know you don't charge this much for delivering a baby, but whenever I remember that you're there, I don't worry that Nora and our baby will be all right. Besides, nobody ever paid you for bringing me into the world, so this hundred dollars is on account. Keep Nora cheerful until I get back.

Love,
JIMMY

Jimmy came back. He and Nora had two other children later, neither of them "on account."

...10

There were many retarded children among these people. This was inevitable, given the intermarriage, the incest, the casual matings throughout the generations. Almost every family had at least one "simple" member. There were also children with physical deformities. One of them, Hester, I sometimes still see in dreams at night. She was the product of her mother and an older brother. She was, by luck, mentally normal, but she was born without legs. I saw her first when, as a child, I went with my mother on one of her calls. We left the car (I think it was Mother's third, a Ford touring car) and started walking up a steep path to the cabin. Hester appeared over the top of the rise, swinging herself down the primitive path with incredible speed on her buttocks with her arms. She was a human pendulum swinging cheerfully toward us, calling greetings. The visits of the woman doctor were precious to her. She had dark curly hair and huge, blazing violet eyes the color of deep amethyst. Hester had fashioned thick deerskin pads for her knuckles and had developed a skill in putting her bottom, without noticeable pause, on spaces in the path without harmful protuberances. When I dream of Hester, even today, I smell violets and acid sour grass, and the thin, sharp scent of young rhododendron leaves motionless in a June sun.

Dr. Nina tried not to interfere with her mountain patients. This must have been hard for her; she was, by temperament, an activist. Whatever happened, her first thought was: What can be done about what has happened? With her special clientele, if she had "done" anything, they would have shut her out and died of the ailments she possibly could alleviate. So she learned to deny herself, to develop enough character to "leave it be," and to have enough faith and trust that in the future, perhaps, she could act to good purpose. But while "leaving it be" with the older persons, she was able to do wonderful things, then and later, for the children.

Dr. Nina always carried with her in her car a bundle of old newspapers. When she entered a shack to deliver a baby she carried her medical bag with one hand and a stack of newspapers with the other. Newsprint is one of the most sanitary materials known to man. Bacteria cannot live on newspaper ink. I suppose new methods of offset printing have destroyed this wonderful property of sterility, but in those days, newsprint was Mother's most dependable ally. She would strip a horrendous bed down to the horrendous mattress, put a thick covering of newspapers under the expectant mother, and deliver a fine, sanitary baby. One time, after the baby had been born and washed and dressed in clothes Dr. Nina had brought with her, the doctor rolled the soiled newspapers and, making a fresh mattress cover of new papers, took the rolled bundle outside to burn it. When she came back into the one-room shack, the new mother furtively thrust something under the covers. Before Dr. Nina had finished making out the birth certificate, smoke began to swirl out of the bed. The woman had taken advantage of a moment of privacy to light up her pipe and then, fearing that the doc might disapprove of pipe smoking, had managed to set her bed on fire. So the doc turned fireman and smothered the fire; she couldn't use water lest she soak the only mattress on the only bed in the cabin. She suggested, mildly, that her patient wait to smoke until the next day, when she could do so out of bed. Another time, she stopped at a cabin on her way back from sewing up a man's leg cut by a glancing blow of an axe. She was checking on a new mother whose baby had been born three days before. She knocked on the door, lifted the latch, and walked in to find the mother nursing a baby skunk. This time Dr. Nina was less mild and very firm.

"But he's an orphan and he's hongry," the woman wailed.

"That's too bad." Dr. Nina was unsentimental. "Your baby needs all the milk you have. You are not ever again to nurse this skunk or anyone else but your baby. Do you understand?"

The woman understood.

One spring day in 1921, Dr. Nina found a note in her mailbox.

Deer Dock. I heerd you was a good docter. I ain't been good since the flew and now I'm terrible sick. I got 3 dollars saved up. Will you come.

GRACE ASHER

Dr. Nina asked around and got directions to the Asher cabin, far back in the hills. The wagon road, almost obscured by new-growth brush, wound up a hill around a stone wall and disappeared. Nina parked the car, took her bag, and walked up a path around a bend, and there, perched on a cliff, was the Asher cabin. Dogs barked and came running down to meet her. Several children swarmed out of the door and ran back in. A lame man limped around the house and out of sight. A woman came to the door and quickly disappeared back inside. Dr. Nina wondered what all the excitement was about. She stopped by the door and looked around. A freshly killed deer lay by the woodpile. No wonder, she thought, they're frightened out of season and out of reason. She laughed at her own pun as she knocked at the now closed door.

Grace Asher, fifteen years old, was very sick indeed. The left side of her chest was thick and swollen; all the breathing she could manage was being done by the right lobes of her lungs.

"Better call your husband," Dr. Nina said to Mrs. Asher. "Grace must go into the hospital immediately. I will need help getting her to the car."

The Monroe County General Hospital had been opened on a shoestring in what had been a large private house in East Stroudsburg. Small and inadequately equipped as it was in the early years, it was much better than many of the places Dr. Nina had to work. Mr. Asher and a neighbor carried Grace to the car on a stretcher Dr. Nina had fashioned out of two poles and an old overcoat. Mrs. Asher followed the doctor to the door as she was leaving.

"We wus scairt when ye come 'cause Dave found a dead deer. We wus goin' to git word to the game warden."

"I wouldn't do that if I were you. Finish skinning it out. Cook it. Eat it. You all need it. Don't worry about me—I didn't see any deer." The two women nodded to each other in perfect understanding.

When Grace came back from the hospital wearing a new dress Dr. Nina had bought for her, the younger children gathered around and looked at their sister with great admiration. Little Harry, five years old, his thin body clad in a cast-off girl's dress, leaned against Dr. Nina's knee.

"Do ye like pheasant?" he asked.

"Why, yes, I do."

"When I git me a gun, I'll shoot one for ye." Harry's face dimpled all over with the idea of such a wondrous gift.

"Bless your heart, Harry! Someday you may just do that."

These two became lifelong friends despite the difference in their ages. Both of them cared about food, both of them all their lives fed the hungry. Harry came to live with us in the fall to go to school. We always had waifs and strays living with us. Mother always found other homes for them as quickly as possible so as to leave room with us for emergency waifs and strays. Harry did well in school. After graduation from high school he won a scholarship to Dartmouth College. He became a world-recognized authority on nutrition, and when Dr. Nina died, many years later, he flew from Italy, where he was a consultant in Rome for the United Nations' Food and Agriculture Organization, to attend her funeral.

...11

In September 1921, when a low-hanging branch ripped loose one of the supports of the Model T's canvas roof and a sharp gust of wind swept the whole top off into the forest, Dr. Nina decided to buy a new automobile. The Dodge agency, the only authorized agency in town at that time, was owned by Arthur M. Price, a handsome, shrewd Welshman, as brave as he was canny. He had given up an important and lucrative position with Armour & Company to risk his future on the future of the horseless carriage. He started with Dodge but later was to become the agent for the Ford Motor Company as soon as Ford was ready to open agencies in the smaller towns.

From the very beginning of our national history, a great many Americans have been nomads. The mass-produced automobile was called into being, evoked, charmed into reality by the wanderlust that is central to the American character. But it took a brave and adventurous mind to believe, the first day the first pleasure car rolled off the assembly line, that this new product would revolutionize the lives of us all. Mr. Price knew from the first that in his lifetime everybody would need to buy a car, and everybody did. He saw in his mind's eye a vast network of fine roads before many roads were even paved. He didn't foresee (and he died before it happened) that our obsession with oil-consuming machines would threaten us all with a nightmare Frankenstein menace of total immobility. Were he here today, he would foresee the future of trains. He was a brave, stalwart, practical, unreconstructed dreamer of the American Dream. He was already what a small town calls "well to do" when Dr. Nina drove in her stripped-down Ford to the A. M. Price garage to buy a new car. She bought a touring car, which is to say an open, canvas-topped sedan with isinglass panels that snapped into place along the sides to keep out the worst of the weather. It was not until her fourth car that the price of closed cars would come within the reach of ordinary people.

A. M. Price allowed Dr. Nina $300 for her old car. She had $200 in cash and arranged to pay off the balance at $40 a month. Mr. Price had never sold a car on credit before; he believed in cash transactions, in closing a deal so that each person could be his own man entirely. The new world of credit buying that was to come and to which he would have to adapt himself never earned his respect. He thought buying on credit was wasteful of money, was sure to undermine self-reliance and independence, and was bad for the country. He never bought anything on credit in his entire life. But for little Dr. Nina he offered credit, not because she had an honest face but because he and Dr. Nina looked at each other and were stricken with love everlasting. Both of them.

I know it's unfashionable these days to talk about falling in love suddenly and totally and forever, but it has happened and probably will happen again in spite of sociological and psychiatric theory. "Now when I passed by thee and looked upon thee, behold, thy time was the time of love." So it was for them. There would be efforts by each one separately to deny the reality of love, but the end was encompassed in the beginning. They were to marry, and their marriage was to last until death parted them more than forty years later.

A. M. took Dr. Nina out for a demonstration spin, and he mentioned, as she drove him back to his office, that he'd heard she often went into the mountains on calls in the evening. He was, he said, always free in the evenings, and would enjoy being her chauffeur. Nina thanked him, but as she drove away she vowed never to see him again. He was a married man, which ruled him out of her future. He refused to stay ruled out. His marriage had been an unhappy one from the start and had been devoid of all sexual encounter for several years. A. M., as everyone called him, was forty-nine years old. His oldest daughter was twenty-three, the next daughter a teenager, and the third a ten-year-old child. From the day he met Dr. Nina, he didn't look back. It was the day his new life began.

Dr. Nina, thirty-six years old, had been separated from

her husband for two years. She decided, finally, to end even the legal remnants of her marriage. She consulted a lawyer about the unknown world of divorce proceedings. It was to be a year later, in the summer of 1922, that she authorized him to prepare for action in the February 1923 term of court. There are no secrets in small towns. Everyone knew Dr. Nina was being driven on out-of-town calls by A. M. Price, that "the woman doctor" was preparing to divorce a minister of the gospel, and that, mark my words, no good would come to her when the excitement of legal proceedings were over. No one could do much to A. M. Price—he had too much money, with the power and respect that money brings in a small town. But Dr. Nina lost most of her paying patients. What the town didn't know then was that A. M. was arranging for an uncontested divorce to be obtained by Nellie, his wife, in return for a very substantial financial settlement.

If I've given the impression that Dr. Nina's medical practice consisted only of mountain patients, I must say now that it is not so. The bulk of her practice was in town and in the outlying farming territory with solid, substantial middle-class people. She had never attracted the elite upper group, for two good reasons. A small-town elite is always conservative-minded and slow to accept social change. A woman doctor was too big a switch from the accepted pattern for the elite to countenance by its patronage. And her fees were modest; elite women have always seen an illogical and snobbish corollary between high fees and good medical treatment. The more a doctor charges, the better doctor he must be. This has not changed, even now. But the attitude of the elite toward Dr. Nina's private life affected the would-be elite, and many of her solid middle-class patients changed to other doctors. The town biddies snubbed her on the street and former patients turned red and stared into shop windows in order not to meet her eye. It was a hard time for Dr. Nina.

But not nearly so hard as the self-righteous had intended. Happiness was no longer a firefly. It was a warm glow in the heart's core, a certainty of mind as complete and as strengthening as the closing of a circle. The beginning of any new thing is always hard, but the beginning of what is believed in inside one's secret self demands only calm fortitude, demands only what the poet Keats once called "negative capability," which is the ability to lean on time, to wait out difficulties, to have, in the words of a popular song of the 1940s, "a little faith and trust in what tomorrow brings." Dr. Nina, who had already practiced negative capability with her mountaineers, was not a slow learner.

...12

Christmas of 1922 was meager in gifts but rich indeed in festivity. Mother had made new doll clothes for each child's favorite doll, and there was one other inexpensive present for each one. The tiny colored lights glowed from inside the rich green of the Christmas tree as softly as stars on a summer night. By ten o'clock in the morning, when Dory Welter, the town's only policeman, rang the bell, the flat was redolent with the aroma of turkey roasting in the oven. Dory was apologetic, but he had been presented with a problem he couldn't solve. A man had come to the police station at the courthouse early Christmas morning. He spoke an unknown tongue but his desperation was evident. Dory had called Tony, the fruit-store man, but the stranger was not speaking Italian; Gus, the shoe repairman, came to help, but the man was not speaking German. No one understood anything. Dory had gone with the stranger to the man's home and had found unpacked suitcases, a small wood fire in the stove, no fire in the coal furnace, no coal, little food, and two beds. In one of them three little girls huddled and in the other the mother shivered with chills and burned with fever. Would Dr. Nina come? She would. Before she left, she telephoned Mr. L'Hommedieu, one of the partners of Zabriskie and L'Hommedieu, Coal and Wood, and persuaded Mr. Man-of-God, a splendid French Catholic, to send a ton of coal and a cord of wood *immediately* to the strangers as a Christmas present.

At the house of the strangers she found no furniture at all except the two beds. As soon as the coal and wood arrived, and the deliverymen had started a good furnace fire and Dr. Nina had built up the fire in the stove, not only in the top of the wood range but also underneath the oven, she walked to the nearest neighbor with a telephone and called Nathan Abeloff, Used Furniture. One might expect that Mr. Abeloff could not easily be persuaded to make a Christmas gift of chairs and a table, but Mr. Abeloff's Jewish heart was as kind as was Mr. L'Hommedieu's and by noon he and his son delivered twelve assorted straight chairs, a table, a rug, and, of all things, two Victorian lamps that a decorator today would pay a fortune to find.

Dr. Nina, with Patrolman Welter in tow, went back to her flat. The policeman carried our Christmas tree, fully trimmed, down the long steep stairway and all the way over to the stranger's house. Mother and Anne Barr packed our Christmas dinner into the touring car along with the three of us, little Harry Asher, and Anne's baby girl. They finished cooking the Christmas dinner at the strangers' house. The tree glowed softly in the warmth. Each of us gave our one meager present to the strangers' little girls, and in spite of the problem of their unknown language we played together all afternoon. Their mother, relieved of the burden of worry and guilt about being unable to cope, which always makes a sick mother sicker, felt better as the hours went by, and that Christmas was as beautiful as any Christmas could ever be. We learned later that the family had come from Czechoslovakia. Why they had arrived in Stroudsburg on Christmas Eve in such a deplorable state of disarray is still unknown to me.

...13

Nellie Price sued for divorce from A. M. Price in the February term of the Monroe County Court. The suit was uncontested. Hints of another woman were given, but no name was mentioned. In a small town, no name needed to be revealed; everybody knew everything—or thought he did. Everyone knew that A. M. Price, properly punished by his wife, would regret his infatuation for the woman doctor and would lead a justly deprived life forevermore. Dr. Nina's suit for divorce was delayed until late in the court term in order that the respondent, Charles Baierle, could attend the hearing, as he wrote that he wished to do. In late April he appeared, listened to Dr. Nina's witnesses, and made the grave error of cross-examining them. Dr. Dorothy Blechschmidt, a throat specialist from Philadelphia, Mame McNeal, Emma Fargo, and others had already given their testimony, all of which the Reverend Charles denied. In his cross-examination of them he only succeeded in eliciting a great deal of new information much more damaging to him than anything they previously had said. It is not wise to bait honest women—their anger is as much to be feared as the anger of the proverbial honest man. Perhaps more to be feared. While being questioned by Dr. Nina's tiny, peppery, brilliant, and partisan lawyer, Ira LeBar, Charles made a pathetic statement. One of the grounds for divorce was nonsupport. Charles had admitted that in their entire marriage he had bought no clothes at all for his wife except for one winter coat years before. Attorney LeBar asked him if he was aware that women cared as much as men for suitable, fashionable clothing. Charles replied, "I don't know much about women." He was boasting, no doubt, of his preoccupation with spiritual matters, but for a married man, the father of three girls, the religious leader of a congregation largely composed of women, such a boast in the dusty, printed record comes across the years as dreary and sad.

On July 2, 1923, Nellie Price was granted a divorce from A. M. Price. On October 6, 1923, Nina Mae Baierle was granted a divorce from Charles Baierle. On October 25, 1923, A. M. Price and Dr. Nina were married.

The town biddies were furious. They had misjudged. That A. M. would marry the "other woman" came as a stunning surprise. That Dr. Nina, who was so unwomanly as to compete with men and was so advanced as to drive a car when everyone knew that only men drove, while ladies sat in the back seat in appropriate apprehension—that such a person should divorce a minister of the gospel and then, instead of suffering, marry the richest man in town caused the ladies to go about grim-faced and tight-lipped. They were to be quite horrid to us all for a few years. Grim respectability is formidable.

But when Mother and Mr. Price arrived back at the flat after their marriage, nothing from outside the family circle intruded on the homecoming. We had planned a gala celebration, but one look at Dr. Nina changed our noisy plans. She was so radiant, so changed in a way we could sense without understanding, so suddenly removed from her previous preoccupation with her children, that we were sobered and confused and immediately respectful of the new day that had dawned for her and thankful that we could go with her into the mysterious world that had made our mother tender and gentle with no fear any more of hidden danger along her way.

PART
SIX

"Rock of Ages, cleft for me,
let me hide myself in thee."

...1

Mother's beloved, A. M. Price, immediately set about to build her a hospital. His hospital was to be much more grandiose than her first one and was, fortunately, of a more flexible design. Should she mean what she said, that she really didn't want to run a hospital, the large three-story brick building could be converted easily into apartments with stores on the ground level. Within two years the conversion was made. The entire second floor was one large apartment for all of us, with Dr. Nina's waiting room and office in the front.

A. M.'s daughters, one by one, came to live with us. No one ever told me why. Their mother had been given their large family home, where she eventually lived alone. Dr. Nina and A. M. had a baby of their own, Catharine, and our home was lively and interesting indeed, with seven girls, many of us near the same age, housekeepers, seamstresses, laundry women, cleaning women, strays, and waifs. A. M. ruled over the entire jumble of humanity without challenge. He had no choice but to become a dictator; with a brilliant and strong-minded wife, one grown daughter, assorted teenagers and preteens, several small children, and a baby, Daddy had to be a dictator or be a cipher. It is inconceivable that such a strong character could drift, by accident, into nothingness.

It is most pleasant to contemplate the marriage of two strong, intelligent persons, both with work to do that engrossed them, and both with such a sense of humor that underneath the discipline that made us into an orderly household ran always a cheerful ripple of laughter.

It was not until after A. M. had lost a great deal of money in the Depression that he became a miser. Perhaps "miser" is too strong a term, carrying with it overtones of greed and selfishness that were no part of A. M. Price's character; but he would not have objected to being called tight-fisted. He rightly concluded that the way to get back the money he had lost was to earn it and not spend it. So he stopped spending money, and Dr. Nina took over paying for everything. Her practice by then was flourishing and she didn't mind spending her money, although she worked long hours for modest fees. She paid the help and the household bills; bought all the food except for random wholesale lots of assorted fruits and meats that A. M. picked up here and there at bargain prices; bought clothes for everyone, including Daddy; paid college bills; gave allowances; bought a new car every two years, giving her old one to Daddy; dressed herself more and more elegantly as time went on, and bought hats and hats and hats, many of them from noted New York designers. She had a good time spending money, and the rest of us had all we needed and more from her warm, generous hands and her warm, merry heart. And with no resentment at all, we respected Daddy's miserliness. It distressed him mightily when Dr. Nina spent her own money for consumer goods that would inevitably wear out. To spare him pain, we all smuggled our purchases into the house while he was at work. I have sometimes said in jest that Daddy never spent a nickel and Mother never told him the truth about money, and their marriage was made in Heaven. Dr. Nina left a modest estate. A. M. died rich. We loved and admired them both. In both their wills, everything was equally divided among the children.

As time went on, the Mrs. Grundys of the town tired of maintaining their self-righteous stances, which were of decreasing effectiveness. Old patients came back and new ones turned up. Other women in Stroudsburg started driving cars and news came in the city papers and over the radio of other women doctors in other places. Little Dr. Nina was no longer a phenomenon to make the town uneasy.

Charles Baierle turned up only one more time in my memory. I was walking home from school the day before we were all to go to court to be legally adopted by A. M. Price. Dr. Nina had no patience with idleness, not even for children. We all learned to read and write when we were three and learned numbers and simple arithmetic when we were four. At five we were ready for school. We usually started in the third grade. So I was very young to deal with such an encounter.

A man had been walking for some time behind the group of little girls I was with on Main Street, long enough for us all to be giving him uneasy glances. He caught up with us and asked if he could speak to me. Remembering Mother's admonition never to speak to strange men, I said no. He said he didn't want to go anywhere, just stand there on the street while we had a few words. He suggested that the other little girls move a few paces down the sidewalk and wait for me. He was persuasive and we agreed.

"Do you know who I am?" he asked.

I didn't know.

"I'm your father."

I was astounded.

He then made an impassioned plea for me to refuse to be adopted. He said, "You will regret it all your life if you allow yourself to become the legal child of a stranger."

How odd it seemed then, when he was the stranger! How odd and how deeply disturbing it was, and how wrong he turned out to be! "The heart knoweth his own bitterness; and a stranger doth not intermeddle with his joy."

...2

Roads were being built as if by magic all over the country and Dr. Nina's mountaineers were exposed to and therefore drawn into the world. She was able to take the state probation officer with her to help her deal with the more nonfunctioning of the backwoods families. A few years before, they would both have been killed for their interference. One family consisted of a senile grandmother, two teenage girls so grievously retarded that they sat all day on the floor of the shack playing with their fingers, their bright blank eyes gleaming behind the long tangled black hair that made veils over their faces, and two young boys under ten years old, one incredibly brilliant, who kept the household barely supplied, and one who appeared to be of marginal intelligence. The grandmother was taken to a nursing home. The two girls were institutionalized. Dr. Nina found a home for the boys with one of her farm families. Both boys, when they grew up, took to farming. Eventually they owned neighboring farms of their own and had their sisters come for a month every summer. The girls, middle-aged by then, played happily all the outdoor children's games their nieces and nephews would simplify for them.

Dr. Nina did not hesitate to remove functioning families from the mountains and into civilization. When she found them caught midway between the past and the future, unwilling to be content with the old and unable to cope with the new, she made a decision for them; she opted for civilization. She was never sentimental about life in the wilderness, I suppose because she knew firsthand how grim a battle it is to survive in partnership only with nature, which is never benign for more than a moment.

One afternoon Dr. Nina was coming from a case at Mud Run when a man stepped out into the road and waited for her car to come to him. She had seen him now and again at neighboring cabins so she knew his name, Adam Vanness, although he had never called her to treat any of his family. He was waiting now to ask her a simple question, but the encounter would lead to a whole new life for the Vannesses. She stopped the car and greeted him.

"Hello, Adam. How are you?"

"I'm all right, but the missus wants fer me to ask if ye have a threwic."

"A threwic? Say that again."

"A threwic," Adam repeated, slowly shaking his head.

"What does she want to do with it?"

"Well, I hate to say it to ye, Doc, but—but she wants somethin' to make her shit." Adam blushed dark red.

"Oh, I see." Dr. Nina was matter-of-fact. "I just couldn't think what she wanted. She wants a physic."

"That's it!" Adam was triumphant. "I knew it was somethin' like that."

While she poured pills into an envelope she asked Adam about his family, and she drove away with an invitation from him to stop back on one of her trips to look over his children.

A few weeks later she walked up a path from the road to their one-room shack. There was a light skif of snow on the ground. The cabin had no window sashes; across the window openings were nailed an assortment of gunnysacks and old blankets. She rapped on the door. It opened and out poured four children, a barking hound dog, and two pigs, one white and one red. Inside, Mrs. Vanness was poking at a smoking stove. Knowing the silent way of these people,

Dr. Nina sat down at the table and looked around. The children and animals came back in again. One of the children fastened the door closed by winding a string around a nail.

"How many of you go to school?" Dr. Nina asked.

"George and Charlie goes," the mother answered. "The rest ain't got no shoes or clothes warm enough. I s'pose ye think it's awful, keepin' pigs in the house, but we hain't got no other place fer 'em and they git cold. They been comin' in and goin' out since they was borned, like the dog, come in and go out, and don't make no mess."

"I never knew you could housebreak a pig." Dr. Nina was smiling and interested. "I learn something new every day!"

The children let her look down their throats and listen to their thin chests. They were fascinated with the stethoscope. Eight-year-old Lillian, with a bright and dimpled face, wore only a man's undershirt with a big tuck held by a safety pin to bring it up to her neck.

"I tell you what, kids," Dr. Nina said. "Next week when I come this way I'll bring some shoes and clothes I've been saving. Maybe we can fit you so you can all go to school."

The children were pathetically eager to find something to fit them in the basket of clothes Dr. Nina brought a week later. Lillian cried when the shoes Dr. Nina had handed her were too small to go on her feet. There was great rejoicing when both shoes and stockings the right size were found. Lillian dimpled all over her face, and the white pig grunted his way from under the bed and stood by the door to be let out.

"Where's the red pig?" Dr. Nina asked.

"We butchered him. We're eating him now. The kids cried," Mrs. Vanness said.

Dr. Nina learned that Adam, the father, was working

every day with his team for a local lumber company. He did all his buying at the company store because he was paid in company scrip, and after he had bought feed for his horses, flour, salt, yeast, sugar, potatoes, and tobacco for himself, he was deeper in debt to the store than the week before. Dr. Nina thought this very strange.

"Tell Adam to ask for a bill for the things he buys this Saturday night, will you, Mrs. Vanness?" Nina asked.

"No use. He don't read."

"Ask him to get the bill for me. I read. And maybe we can figure out a way for you to get more out of a week's work."

She checked the bills from week to week and found that Adam was being charged exorbitant prices. She assumed that the cheating was the work of the company store clerk, and with the best will in the world she made an appointment with one of the partners in the company. She showed him Adam's receipts and a comparative list of prices from the cash stores in the area. The partner exploded in resentment. He advised the doctor to mind her own business. He told her what he thought of interfering females. He had a rough tongue.

The partner was running for state senator from that district. Wherever Dr. Nina went for the next six weeks she told her voting patients her little tale of the partner's refusal to interest himself in simple honesty and justice. He lost the election.

She found a job in Stroudsburg for Adam and a house on the outskirts of town. The children, George, Charlie, Lillian, and Chester, all did well in life and Dr. Nina delivered their babies and their grandchildren.

The mountain settlements were breaking apart. Some of the men and some of the young women walked out of the woods to a new road and walked away into oblivion. With

Dr. Nina's help, other families moved closer to town. Whenever she found some sprout of intelligence in a mountain child, she arranged for him to go to school; if the home were unsuitable and not capable of being reorganized, he lived with us until a permanent home could be found. Those who stayed in the hills found work on the roads or at the paper mill, and with cash money to do with and electric power lines following the new highways to tap into, they rebuilt their shacks into houses with town conveniences. They began to pay the doctor and to take pride in paying.

One day a young mountain boy walked into the office.

"How much do ye charge to born a baby?"

"That depends," Dr. Nina replied, "upon where it is and who it is. Who's going to have a baby?"

"My ma. She ain't never had no doctor for none of us, but I work now and I want for her to have a doctor."

"How much money do you have?" Dr. Nina asked.

"I got fifteen dollars saved. Will that be enough?" he asked fearfully.

"Yes, indeed. That's just right. You're a fine boy to do this for your mother. I'll come whenever you need me."

"I come after ye now," he said.

Dr. Nina went.

...3

The waifs and strays who lived with us over the years were a mixed bag of unfortunates. Often they were children, but sprinkled among them were pregnant girls whose families, pillars of one church or another, had cast them out when their mistake was evident. Dr. Nina always, with discretion, talked to the boys involved, themselves sons of church pillars. Surprisingly enough, many of the boys were eager to marry, to "do the right thing"; it was only ineptitude and fear of the parents that stood in the way of a solution. In those cases Dr. Nina herself talked to the parents, and the marriages that resulted were as happy as most. Where no marriage was possible or desirable, the girl lived with us until the birthing and the return to good health. If the girl was determined not to keep the baby, Dr. Nina found a good home suitable to the child's background, a personal history Dr. Nina knew a thousand times more thoroughly than any forms could reveal in a placement agency. Today I watch those of her babies that I know with the pride and satisfaction of an aunt by adoption.

When the baby was safely placed, Dr. Nina turned her blue, concentrated gaze on the young mother. She found a place for the girl to live, a job, a new life in a new environment, a new opportunity to "walk proud" in self-respect. I can't estimate how many times she left no stone unturned until the need of a young person was met.

The children who lived with us were so numerous that I've forgotten many of them. I do remember the twins. Dr. Nina was called too late that time. By the time she reached the remote farm in the west end of the county, the premature twins had been born, their cords tied and cut, and the mother had bled her life away through a retained placenta. Theirs was a good family of Pennsylvania Dutch stock, but evil times had come upon them. The father had been killed in his own field by a stupid, careless hunter, and the mother, dazed by grief, had paid no heed to her own state of health until there was no health at all. The fire in the stove had been banked for the night, but there was some warmth left. Dr. Nina washed and wrapped the babies and tucked them in the oven until she could comfort the oldest daughter, get the other three children to bed, clean up the mess, and fetch a neighbor to stay the rest of the night. She brought the twins home.

Responsible kin took the four older children after the funeral, but no one would take the premature twin boys. They lived and thrived. We had them for nine months because Dr. Nina felt that twins should stay together and she could find no adopting family that would take them both. Finally and reluctantly, she decided to separate them in order to make room at our house for the Burton boys, whose need was dire. The two sets of new parents were poles apart in their ideas of how to raise adopted children. One twin was taken by a railroad engineer and his wife who were leaving town to live in the city at the other end of his railroad run.

"No one in that place will know he's not our child," they said. "When we return here in three or four years, every-one will think he was born while we were away. We'll raise him as our own and never tell him he's adopted." They left town in great secrecy one night after stopping for the baby and smuggling him out of the house as one smuggles a fabulous gem to safety.

The other twin went to a pressman and his wife. They sent out announcements. They had a christening party with all their friends. They said, "We believe a child should grow up with the knowledge that he's adopted, that we chose him for our own. Then he can never be shocked or hurt if he finds it out later."

Three years passed. The engineer, his wife, and the baby returned to Stroudsburg and moved into one side of a dou-ble house on a quiet, pleasant street. The next morning Billy was sent out into the yard to play. His mother, hear-ing him talking to someone and hearing another child's voice piping back, went out on the porch. Almost at the same moment, the next-door neighbor came out on her porch. One look at the two boys and both women stared at each other with astonishment.

"So you took the other twin!" they exclaimed in unison.

In her long medical practice, Dr. Nina saw the results of many cases of child abuse, most of them ending in death. The abuse of children is a most heinous crime, all the more frightful because the abuser is out of his own control. No sane person tortures a child. It is a dreadful aberration that knows no one country, no one social class, no one fixed and recognized method of operation. And the commission of this crime is usually impossible to prove.

Dr. Nina took every suspicion to the authorities, who, with regret, refused to bring charges that could be proved only by the legally unacceptable inferences of a professional mind. In the case of the Burton boys, she took action by herself, and a great deal of time and trouble were to be spent before she found a happy solution for them.

Harold, nine years old, and Stanley, seven, had been legally adopted by Mary and Ed Lenear after the Burtons, neighbors of the Lenears, had died in the flu epidemic. The adoption must have been Ed's idea, for Mary was unfit as a parent. She could stand Harold, who had learned quickly how to cope with her, but Stanley's fear of her enraged her until she had spiraled out of control into vicious hatred. He was subjected to cruel whipping. Both boys were seriously undernourished, but Stanley was close to actual starvation. As soon as Ed left for work, Mary chained Stanley in a cold outdoor shed, with only a piece of rag rug to lie upon. She brought him in before Ed came home and beat him so that he would be sobbing woefully. This constant crying did not endear him to Ed.

Dr. Nina came upon this dreadful situation by chance and persuaded Mary to let her take both boys home with her. Stanley was very sick; one ear was badly infected, his temperature was high. Dr. Nina was shocked anew when she bathed the little boys and saw the scars on Stanley's matchstick body. She put Harold to bed and took Stanley into the kitchen, where she put warm drops in his ear and, with a hot-water bottle between his ear and her chest, rocked him in a big rocker and sang him to sleep.

The next morning she heard the boys talking.

"What did the doc do to you in the kitchen? Did she whip you?" Harold asked.

"No. She put something in my ear. She rocked me. She sang a song about a kitty. She was just like a mother!"

I wonder how the poor little tyke knew what a mother was like.

A brisk three-week battle ensued with Ed Lenear. He was sure there must be a reason why Dr. Nina wanted the boys, and the only reason he could imagine was that she'd found out the boys were heirs to a fortune from some unknown source. The battle became a bit rowdy at times, with lawyers shouting at each other in Dr. Nina's waiting room. Ed Lenear was on the verge of victory when Mary announced that even with the court order for the return of the boys she would never have them in the house again. The battle collapsed. We won the Burton boys.

It was a victory, but not an unmixed one. For a few weeks still they cowered in corners, whimpered in their sleep, dodged if a hand reached toward them, but then the healthier and happier the boys became, the livelier and more inventive their games grew to be. The house, and especially the plumbing, was often in shambles during the year they lived with us. The thin, sparce bristle-like hair that had sprouted from their tiny skulls when they first arrived grew long and shining. A. M. became the haircutter, and with scissors and clippers kept them looking like civilized children. Their eyes, which had looked so enormous in their thin tiny faces, shrank to normal size as their cheeks rounded. Their energy never flagged. We were not entirely sad when Dr. Nina found the right home with the right family for the Burton boys.

... 4

Because of Dr. Nina's rejection of idleness, her children graduated from college at an early age. We all married young, but not too young, as it turned out, to know what we were doing. Life began to be easier for the doctor. Her practice grew and grew and the money was more and more her own. Instead of buying Ford cars, she advanced briefly to Mercurys and then, in a great leap forward, to Lincolns. She had always dreamed of driving a Lincoln Continental the way others dream of owning a Degas or wearing diamonds. As soon as she could afford it, she bought a new Lincoln every two years, usually special-order pink. Dr. Nina's pink Linc was always in demand by the city fathers to cart VIP guests around the area. The elite of the town women suddenly discovered what everyone else had known for years, that Stroudsburg, Pennsylvania, had a Natural Wonder that the outside world was beating a path to the town to consult. Patients were coming regularly from Scranton, Allentown, Harrisburg, Philadelphia, New York. They came because the word had spread far and wide that there was a doctor in Stroudsburg who could find out what was really the trouble; who had a talent, a sixth sense for diagnosis. I think what we all want most from a doctor is a definition of the problem, a clear statement of what has gone wrong either with our complicated bodies or our even more complicated minds.

A new day was dawning for women in our world and in my home town. The local college began to hire women professors. Women opened specialty shops and became real-estate and insurance agents. Soon there were enough financially independent women to form a Business and Professional Women's Club, and Dr. Nina, the outcast, became a happy, enthusiastic, and charming member of this new and envied elite. It must have been fun for her, especially in view of her personal philosophy that each day was a new day to be glad in; that the hater always suffers more than the hated; that anger and leftover grudges literally poison the cells of the mind. So she could enter a new era with the past wiped out totally.

The Monroe County Medical Association, which had ignored this member for years except to be amused at her wondrous hats, asked her to organize a child health committee; she did, and was a member of the Executive Committee from then on, and served as vice president and president whenever she was needed. She was elected president of the Stroudsburg Business and Professional Women's Club and went to the state convention. For most of us, that a club convention could be a marvelous event would be unthinkable. For Dr. Nina, new as a wide-eyed baby to any convention, it *was* marvelous. She went armed with a sheaf of resolutions from her local chapter, and when the convention was ended, the other delegates went back to their counties with unaccustomed hope that their organization was entering a new era of effectiveness in the life of the state. It probably was.

Every Wednesday A. M. Price went to the Penn Stroud Hotel for the luncheon of the Stroudsburg Kiwanis Club, and Dr. Nina gave herself the modest treat of lunching out at Wyckoff's Tearoom. She would take one of us, whoever was around at the moment, or meet friends there for lunch, as pleased with the outing as though the tearoom were Sardi's or 21. Word soon spread that Dr. Nina could be found at the tearoom at noon on Wednesday, and patients from the country in for a day's shopping would gather to ask for a quick prescription for someone ailing at home, joined by Wyckoff's Department Store employees with their minor ailments of the moment, and by everyone else who, attracted by the crowd, seized the opportunity to discuss small physical or family problems with Dr. Nina. Ernest Wyckoff, Sr., was the merchandising genius who founded this excellent store. (I still shop there, and at other shops as well, Smith's, Burrows', Vi's, for clothes that I wear to events here and in Europe. A gown from Vi's brought a gracious compliment from Emilio Pucci himself at a dinner party in Florence.) Mr. Wyckoff put a rueful and humorous ad in the *Pocono Record* (formerly the Stroudsburg *Daily Record*) noting that Dr. Nina's Wednesday patients made it appear that the tearoom was having a weekly anniversary sale. He suggested that Dr. Nina's following, after the free consultations, might enjoy sitting at the tearoom tables for the Wednesday special.

As time passed, a river of better paying patients came to Dr. Nina. Among the more affluent elite who turned to her and never turned away again was the Fisher family of Swiftwater, a mountain resort near Stroudsburg. That family, which lived a rigid and exclusive life on inherited money in a great old house whose back porches were cantilevered out over a forest gorge, consisted of an ancient, autocratic mother, upright and slender as a spring sapling but with a temperament unyielding as an oak; Bessie, a fifty-plus-year-old daughter, dressed in the old style with skirts that swept the floor; and Esther, forty-five, the modern sister who, in a Girl Scout leader's uniform that stopped halfway between knee and ankle, did Good Works and ran the entire county Girl Scout organization with an efficient, dedicated, firm hand.

Bessie was an intellectual. She studied insects and had marvelous equipment, microscopes and slides and laboratory fittings of such diversity that it was a pleasure for any of us to go with Mother to the Fisher home just to stand admiringly at the door of Bessie's workroom. We liked the house, too; nothing had been changed inside for eighty years. But best of all we admired Bessie's mustache, which was thick and gray and unabashed to find itself on the face of a beskirted bluestocking. Soon we had something even better to look at: Bessie's apes.

They were two chimpanzees that had apparently been abandoned by one of the small traveling circuses that roamed the country in those days. Bessie had spotted them swinging from the tops of the trees that met the cantilevered porch. She stocked up on bananas and fed them daily, luring them bit by bit closer to the house. A carpenter, meanwhile, had been employed to construct giant cages, reinforced with iron, on the porch. Bessie lured the apes up to the porch and into the cages and closed and locked the doors. She opened up one of the unused rooms in the big house and furnished a new laboratory with wonderful new equipment for the study of primates. Then she set herself the task of taming and making friends with the apes.

The apes refused to cooperate. No matter how cunningly and resourcefully she tried to win their trust, they bit her. The Fisher family had, none of them, ever sat in a doctor's waiting room; the doctor, naturally, came to them. Dr. Nina was called once a week, on the average, to check the health of the three women, but after the apes were caged, Dr. Nina came almost every other day to bind up Bessie's wounds. The interesting thing was that the Fishers never paid her a cent. At her first visit Mrs. Fisher informed Dr. Nina that she expected "professional courtesy." Her husband, dead for many years, had been a doctor, and it was only right that no doctor should charge for services to another doctor's family. Extremes do meet. The poor without a cent to give and the rich without a cent to waste have much in common. In another sense, Dr. Nina was paid; at the Fisher house she met their sister-in-law, Dorothy Canfield Fisher, who accompanied their brother on occasional visits to the family home. It was Dorothy Canfield who, fascinated and entranced by Dr. Nina, convinced her that she should make notes on her professional life so that this era of our national history would not be lost.

...5

After Dr. Nina and A. M.'s household had shrunk to the two of them, except for waifs and strays, together they began a study and collection of minerals. They took a summer off to wander across the country to California with metal detectors and Geiger counters to gather rocks and prospect for uranium. At an age when other couples totter around the neighborhood for exercise, Dr. Nina, over sixty, and A. M., over seventy, prospected in the deserts of the West and fished the icy streams of the Rockies. They visited us in Rome. It was their first trip to Europe and their first jet ride. We watched the oxen plow the country fields in Umbria, ate pasta and drank ice-cold white wine in Piazza Navona, toured Pompeii, dined on octopus and garlic-stuffed artichoke hearts at Terracina while watching the fishing boats set out over the slate-gray evening sea. We did everything they wanted to do, and it was a busy three

weeks. A. M. was impressed with the only country he'd
ever seen outside of North America. "These Italians are
coming back!" he said.

A new element had been added to Dr. Nina's vigorous
practice of medicine: the role of consultant. As she approached her fiftieth year of medical practice, she had already seen many rare diseases, many unusual complications, many ordinary ailments so masked by secondary
problems as to be unrecognizable from textbook descrip-
tions. One day in 1956 she was called to the new, fully
equipped Monroe County General Hospital to consult
with a young doctor about a patient of his who was very
sick but whose symptoms seemed to add up to a disease
unknown to the human race. I waited in a wide, spotless
corridor while Mother examined the patient. She came out
of the room saying to the doctor, "I know that's what it is,
because I had a case just like this in 1912. I was baffled then,
too. The reason it's so difficult to diagnose . . ." and she
began a medical explanation much too complicated for me
to follow. I was amused. The young doctor could not even
have been born in 1912. It should have been edifying for
him to watch Dr. Nina, her white hair peeping out from
under the mass of roses on her hat, her white doctor's coat
stiff and starched, turn her light-blue, concentrated gaze on
the patient, and, rejecting false evidence, shut out the
whole world while she searched for medical truth in a
human body that was, for her, not an object but a person
who deserved respectful treatment.

In her own practice she was delivering the third generation of babies, having remarkable success in her own
method of treating arthritis, helping to found a locally
supported home for the indigent aged, seeking help for
children, counseling young persons, and everywhere sharing openly and unself-consciously her certainty that any-

body could do anything that was required of him. To anyone who said to Dr. Nina, "I can't stand it," her firm answer came back, "Of course you can."

...6

In 1957 the celebration of Dr. Nina's fiftieth year in practice got under way. The most formal celebration was a gala luncheon in Harrisburg put on by the state medical society, with the president of the American Medical Association and the governor of Pennsylvania attending. The most pleasant event was the dinner in Stroudsburg arranged by the Monroe County Medical Society. The dinner was unpublicized. "It had to be that way," said one of the speakers, "otherwise there would not be a place large enough to hold all the people who would want to come." So only a few hundred people were invited. Dr. Nina thought she was going out for dinner with her family, and when she was squired to the ballroom entrance and saw such an array of her colleagues and friends, she said, "There must be some mistake. We've come to the wrong place. There's some sort of formal dinner going on here." There was indeed. Seconds later, Dr. Nina was among them, a slim white-haired figure in a pink chiffon gown, and as she was shepherded along, she was filled with wonder. The wonder grew as she was led the full length of the ballroom and the crowd stood for fully five minutes cheering and clapping. Throughout the dinner hour, clapping broke out again from time to time as diners exchanged anecdotes about the honored guest. Dr. Nina made a charming response to all the laudatory speakers. She was funny and touching and intelligent. For twenty minutes she told stories. She was as unself-

conscious and as graceful as though she were holding spell-
bound her own family.

"I don't know," she concluded, "why you feel I've done
so much and not been repaid. I've had more fun in my work
than I could ever have had in any other field. I've been
repaid a thousand times—by little babies who grew up to
be strong men and women and good citizens, and by men
and women who not only have thanked me in a million
ways, but who are my friends." Dr. Nina was seventy-three
years old.

The most amusing sidelight on her celebration year came
when the doctor in charge of a reception being planned for
her by the Women's Medical College in Philadelphia called
my sister Bobby to ask if "Dr. Nina could still get around
by herself." That morning Bobby had arranged to meet Dr.
Nina in Allentown for some shopping. They were to meet
at the elevators of the largest department store. Dr. Nina
had hurried in, late, and after the elevator doors had closed
said to Bobby, "I'm sorry I'm late. I had twins at three
o'clock this morning, and a miscarriage at six." Not a sound
was made as all the shoppers turned to look at Dr. Nina.
The elevator door slid silently open and shut for the second
floor before those who had intended to get off recovered
from their surprise at such a statement from a white-haired
woman who blushed and twinkled, merry-eyed, under
their gaze. Bobby assured the doctor from Philadelphia
that Dr. Nina could dance a jig around the latest graduates
of her institution.

In 1960 Dr. Nina was featured abroad by the United
States Information Service as an example of a successful
American woman who had gained recognition in a profes-
sional sphere. The copy of the feature article we sent her
from Yugoslavia, in Serbo-Croatian and written in the
Cyrillic alphabet, made her laugh.

In 1962 Dr. Nina was named Pennsylvania Woman of the Year. The nomination was entered jointly by the Business and Professional Women's Club and the Soroptimist Club, and letters of support poured into Harrisburg. The testimonials from men's organizations (the Kiwanis Club, Lions, Chamber of Commerce, Exchange Club, Medical Society, and so on) tended to stress her unpaid services. Her male colleagues estimated that she had been paid by less than 40 percent of her patients, and the men in the community were impressed and indeed bemused by such benevolence. The women's organizations stressed her accomplishments, not just the ones we know about, but (from the Business and Professional Women's Club) "Dr. Nina organized clinics for young women in all phases of hygiene, but particularly in prenatal care and care of the child"; and (the Red Cross) "She was a pioneer in the cancer crusade in the county"; and (the Visiting Nurse Association) "There were many occasions when Dr. Nina would recruit people to visit with the isolated and the lonely. Many of these visits evolved themselves into songfests and happy parties. A cheerful environment was of great therapeutic value in the treatment of these patients."

Churches of all denominations wrote, Methodist, Baptist, Episcopal, Catholic. The pastor of the Presbyterian church, in which all of Dr. Nina's children were raised, wrote, "Only the annals of eternity will reveal the number of lives she has touched and the number of homes she has helped. We have come to expect that our doctors will be self-sacrificing and benevolent. Dr. Nina, however, has stretched this expectation almost beyond belief." Hundreds of her patients wrote. It must have become a town project to take some part, no matter how small, in the general outpouring of gratitude. One patient wrote a one-sentence letter: "I shall never forget that she comes right over when you call her each time." Another wrote two sentences: "She could always be counted on when you needed her most, which was life-saving to the people in the country who couldn't get to town. Dr. Nina has delivered many children in her career as doctor, and money, whether you had it or not, was no object to her."

It was all very beautiful.

...7

Dr. Nina closed her medical practice in 1964 to have more time for her ailing ninety-two-year-old husband. A. M. Price had had a heart attack, three small strokes, and now had cancer. He died in November 1966, quietly, without complaint, and in severe and total dignity. "So let us melt, and make no noise." Eighty-two-year-old Dr. Nina then had a massive stroke and went to live in a nursing home in State College, Pennsylvania, where her second daughter, Carol, lived with her Pennsylvania State University professor husband.

Dr. Nina had said many times that when she could no longer work, and if she had to live without Daddy, she would fall apart like the one-horse shay and be no more. But the mind and the will do not decide such things; another force takes over, a life force, a will to live that comes from the hidden depths of the secret cells. She recovered enough from the stroke to begin a new life that was wounded and circumscribed but a new life, nevertheless.

One of her private nurses was a pretty young woman whose training had been in nursing care for children. Her skill, her intelligence, and her gentle, pleasing personality were so impressive that Carol persuaded her to try geriatric nursing. She began on Monday, and on Tuesday she called Carol.

"I can't do this," she said. "I'm sorry, but I can't work where there is no hope." She agreed to stay on until Carol could find a replacement.

On Friday she called again.

"Carol, if you haven't hired someone else, I'd like to stay. I've changed my mind, because there *is* hope."

A second nurse, Janet Packard, was a blessing to us all. Had she been Dr. Nina's own child, she could not have been more loving or more full of grace. She was with Dr. Nina until the end.

A third nurse did leave after two years to enter medical school. She'd always wanted to be a doctor but had never before had the courage to begin. Dr. Nina had that effect on people, sharing as she did Socrates' opinion that "he is not only idle who does nothing; he is also idle who might be better employed." She had absolute faith in the potential of any person willing and brave enough to try new paths. "They go from strength to strength, every one of them."

On her ninetieth birthday, all the furniture except her bed had to be moved from her room to make space for the guests who came with flowers and presents. There was champagne and Dr. Nina, pink and white as a crumpled rose, drank a sip after the toasts and promptly closed her eyes and slept away the celebration, smiling faintly in her sleep.

On a June day in 1974, Dr. Nina died.

If there is a Heaven, Dr. Nina is surely there, and I think there are no panthers in heaven. I can see her now as she turns her energies to her new work in the Elysian fields. I fancy that just inside the Pearly Gates she has set up a dispensary complete with a neat brass sign that says:

Dr. Nina's Dispensary
Free Consultations
Young People a Specialty

And I can see her looking over the frightened young souls of those whose lives were cruelly interrupted by war, by illness, by accident, or by the folly that others, given more time, lived to correct. And if, as she said many years before, God sees us not as we are but as we would have been if love and luck had blessed us all, then she is looking over groups of souls as variegated as armloads of wild flowers gathered in a spring wilderness in Pennsylvania—violets, wild ladyslippers, snowdrops, and trailing arbutus, whose heavenly scent quivers the very leaves that hide its shy white flowers.

And I can hear her now as she goes from group to group, saying:

"Don't be lazy.

"Put in honest time.

"Decide how much time you can give to becoming the best of all angels, and if at first the work seems hard, don't be discouraged.

"Excellence follows honest work.

"Do with your might what your hands find to do.

"The Lord has made room for you."